PRAISE

"*Stellar Sex* is an incredibly fun a _____ _____ intimacy and self-love through the lens of astrology. It opens doors to rewrite the narratives we have around sex and vulnerability while remaining engaging. Aubrey does an excellent job taking us through our own charts to help identify what may work for us…and what may not. She expertly showcases the gifts and shadows of each placement, allowing us to delve deeper into our own psyches. She reminds us that it isn't just about the relationship we have with the planets or the relationship we have with others, but more the relationship we have with ourselves. Real intimacy comes from within."

—ANTHONY PERROTTA, astrologer

"*Stellar Sex* offers a holistic view of intimacy, whether it's the most receptive areas of the body based on one's astrological placements or the words needed to get in the mood. Aubrey Houdeshell is a talented writer who demystifies astrology for novices and gives those with experience something new to consider. You'll find yourself flipping through repeatedly to learn about yourself, your lovers, crushes, and more in this fascinating introduction to sextrology!"

—STERLING MOON, author of *Talking to Spirits*

"In this beginner-friendly foray into sextrology, Aubrey validates readers' most private desires, bolstering self-awareness and self-confidence. *Stellar Sex* is a clear, accessible look at how planets, asteroids, and other natal placements contribute to our needs in intimate relationships. With Aubrey's expert guidance, readers will learn how to look at the sum of their birth chart's parts to live a truly satisfying life."

—NICOLE WELLS, author of *It's All About Astrology*

STELLAR
SEX

ABOUT THE AUTHOR

Aubrey Houdeshell is a writer, astrologer, and lover of all things ethereal. Her work focuses mainly on the transformative and healing potential contained within the exploration and knowledge of the self. Her other works include the *Oracle of Pluto* and *The Cosmic Symposium*. She lives in Denver with her husband and family. Visit her on Instagram at @AubreyCHoudeshell.

STELLAR SEX

UNLOCK YOUR SEXUAL POWER WITH EROTIC ASTROLOGY

AUBREY HOUDESHELL

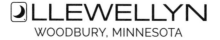

LLEWELLYN
WOODBURY, MINNESOTA

First Edition
First Printing, 2025

Book design by Donna Burch-Brown
Cover design by Shira Atakpu

Llewellyn Publications is a registered trademark of Llewellyn Worldwide Ltd.

Library of Congress Cataloging-in-Publication Data (Pending)
ISBN: 978-0-7387-8020-7

Llewellyn Worldwide Ltd. does not participate in, endorse, or have any authority or responsibility concerning private business transactions between our authors and the public.

All mail addressed to the author is forwarded but the publisher cannot, unless specifically instructed by the author, give out an address or phone number.

Any internet references contained in this work are current at publication time, but the publisher cannot guarantee that a specific location will continue to be maintained. Please refer to the publisher's website for links to authors' websites and other sources.

Llewellyn Publications
A Division of Llewellyn Worldwide Ltd.
2143 Wooddale Drive
Woodbury, MN 55125-2989
www.llewellyn.com

Printed in the United States of America

OTHER BOOKS BY AUBREY HOUDESHELL

The Cosmic Symposium:
An Astrological Journey Through
the Orchestra of the Planets
(Illustrated by Rose Ides,
Running Press, 2024)

Oracle of Pluto:
A 55-Card Exploration of
the Undiscovered Self
(Illustrated by Rose Ides,
RP Studio, 2023)

This book is dedicated to the lover in all of us.
To the heart that burns and burns and burns.

CONTENTS

THIRD BASE: TAKING THINGS A STEP FURTHER

INTRODUCTION

The intersection of sex and astrology, known as *sextrology*, is something I have centered my practice around for a handful of years now. Sex is a fundamental part of life and is something I've seen many people, including myself, struggle to have a healthy, empowered relationship with, especially when it comes to truly understanding our own erotic nature. What are our wants, needs, and desires? How does our erotic energy wish to express itself? How can we honor this part of ourselves in a truly authentic way? These are questions that can feel elusive to many of us for any number of reasons, but certainly in part because of the messages society still sends, even in our modern age.

As somebody with their own sexual trauma, I have certainly struggled with sexuality, and it can be difficult to find avenues to explore all that it encompasses in a way that feels safe and free of shame. That's where astrology comes in.

The birth chart is an invaluable tool for knowing ourselves. It truly encompasses the entirety of the human experience, from creativity to love, money, family, travel, and so on. So, I thought, why not sex?

At the inception of my exploration into the sexual birth chart, I started with the obvious placements: Venus and Mars (the two partnership planets) and the eighth house (which, as we will see, is the house of sex). Through both exploring my own chart (which contains plenty of overtly sexual energies) and giving readings tailored specifically to sexual expression, my view on the erotic energies of the chart began to expand, until it became clear to me that every single piece of the chart can be used to deepen our understanding of

1

the eroticism that courses through each of our beings, bodies, minds, hearts, and souls. Thus, the idea for *Stellar Sex* was born.

My experience of writing this book was an interesting one. Though I've never been someone who is scandalized by sex or anything surrounding it the way many others seem to be, I am also someone who is quite private in this area—you can thank my Scorpio Venus for that, I suppose. I've never been one to kiss and tell, nor to divulge the nitty-gritty of my sexual escapades the way some of my friends do. There's nothing wrong with that, of course. It's just not who I am. So when it came time to sit down and start talking about sextrology, I had to determine the best way to approach this topic.

All that is to say, this book is not a how-to. While there are suggestions on some things to try in order to really honor the planetary energies in a chart, this book is more about understanding the wants and needs of your chart through a sexual lens. Thanks largely to my Virgo Mercury in the twelfth house, I believe that a key component of the spiritual journey involves real, tangible examples and understanding. Since Mercury rules over writing, that is the way this book is written. *Stellar Sex* is more of an introductory book than anything else, a jumping-off point. My goal is to give you the tools and understanding you need about your sexual side so that you can go out and have the real experiences you're craving in your connections with others. I also don't believe in telling people what to do, and I certainly don't believe in trying to define anyone's sexuality. We are our own sovereign beings in that regard, and the best way I can see to honor that, and to facilitate the process of self-knowledge, understanding, and empowerment, is to let you decide how best to harness the information herein.

Life is inherently relational. As human beings, we are hardwired to need one another, and as a result, every facet of our lives is made up of relationships. We are in relationship with one another, whether as friends, family members, professional connections, or lovers. We have relationships with nature, with money, with the stars in the sky, with our bodies, and, perhaps most importantly, with ourselves. There is nothing we do that exists in a vacuum; whether we realize it or not, we are always interacting with something. Even seemingly inconsequential things are laced with the mysterious divine intelligence that courses through the fabric of the universe. Even empty vessels are made of *something*. And thus, the importance of understanding ourselves—our wants, needs, and desires—is a crucial element of being able to successfully navigate every facet of our lives. Through the age-old adage "Know thyself," we can come to find empowerment and can successfully move out into the world and begin to create a life of fulfillment. There are, of course, innumerable avenues through which we can come to understand ourselves better, but the one I've come to explore and know the most is astrology.

Astrology is something that has been practiced for millennia, with some of the earliest evidence of it dating as far back as the third millennium BCE. The study of astrology is deeply intertwined with human history, with some kind of astrological practice present in cultures across the globe. For a long time, up until about the seventeenth century, it was considered a traditional academic pursuit. While the space that astrology takes up in today's culture is much different, it remains a point of interest and study that transcends the boundaries of class and culture.

Ultimately, astrology fascinates us because it reveals the relationship between the planets moving in the sky and human affairs down here on Earth. Each one of us has our own personal map, commonly known as the birth chart or natal chart, that is calculated using the exact time and place of birth and that, when studied, offers incredible insight into our individual nature and life. Learning the ins and outs of our birth chart can help us to understand the great complexities of what it means to be human and the role we're playing in the microcosm of our life, as reflected in the movements of the heavenly bodies of the macrocosm. As above, so below, as the saying goes.

People also get into astrology because it's *fun*.

There are arguably more people paying attention to astrology now than ever before. Thanks to social media, astrologers and spiritual practitioners are reaching millions of people, and astrological phenomena such as the infamous Mercury retrograde have shot astrology into the limelight, garnering an insane amount of popularity and traction. We can see astrology's influence everywhere, from brand accounts to articles, television shows, and products. Pop culture is turning to astrology in greater and greater swaths, with no end in sight. This trend echoes a greater sentiment within the collective consciousness that points to people's desire to know themselves and to find empowerment within that search.

The same can be said for sex.

Sex is often credited with being the oldest industry in existence. Just like astrology, sex is deeply intertwined in human history—arguably more so than anything else, as it is the reason humans continue to exist at all. As complex, and perhaps taboo, as the topic of sex may be, it is a fundamental part of being a person and a fundamental part of relationships. And, just like astrology, sex is everywhere.

I find some people's reactions to sex to be quite funny. Even in today's age, despite the ongoing sexual revolution fueled by things like hookup culture and the ever-increasing number of dating apps, there are those who are scandalized by even the mention of sex. Why? Because there still exists a dark underbelly around sex that is rooted in shame and fear. There are still those who pedal the idea that sex and all its animalistic urges are some kind of sin or trick or outside force that acts upon us and needs to be rejected or controlled or stamped out. And as much as some people might like to tell themselves that they've moved past those messages, we can still see their sinister influence poking through in people's visceral reactions to sex.

As somebody who was raised Catholic and was taught abstinence through a scary and highly graphic slideshow of sexually transmitted diseases in middle school, I have firsthand knowledge of the anti-sex bullshit that still gets force-fed to our youth. And yet, despite the efforts of many terrified adults in my life, I have always been a very sexually confident person (probably thanks largely to my Leo South Node, but more on that later). I have never really understood why people are so scandalized by pretty much anything related to sex—who is having it and with whom, sex work, people's varying sexual identities, and so on—especially since it's something that most of us engage in. I am an ardent supporter of a more realistic, inclusive sex education. I believe that knowledge is power, and it is only through being given the tools we need to make informed choices that we are able to approach sex and everything it encompasses in a truly healthy, empowering way.

It is from this belief that *Stellar Sex* was born. The intention behind this book is to grant the gift of knowledge and understanding and to help demystify the sometimes abstract and downright complicated nature of astrology that can leave people feeling overwhelmed and confused. Through unraveling all the nuances of the various influences of the planets in the chart, and how they influence love, romance, and sex, we can begin to understand our erotic selves. This initiation, then, offers us the chance to name and give life to the parts of us that are full of desire, lust, and need. We can unlock the deep passion in our hearts and move toward pleasure, intimacy, and, ultimately, love. My hope is that, through the *Stellar Sex* journey, you can begin to honor and revere the passionate creature within and find union with these parts of yourself through understanding—and have a good time doing it.

WHAT IS SEXTROLOGY?

Sextrology is exactly what it sounds like: sex through the lens of astrology. Truly, it is the art of unraveling our sexual and romantic nature: our approach to romantic and/or sexual connections, our wants and desires, what turns us on and off, the things we value, and our larger needs for sex and intimacy as a whole. With sextrology, we can learn about the way we express these desires, the way we express our sexuality, and our must-haves and deal-breakers, as well as how to embody the energy of our astrological placements to amp up our own personal brand of magnetism.

By studying our birth chart through the lens of sextrology, we can find potent magick, healing, and deeper fulfillment in ourselves, our relationships, and possibly our lives as a whole. When we educate ourselves on these aspects of our loved ones as well, we can learn how to be better partners, lovers, and friends. Remember that relationships are a two-way street (or more, if you practice any form of nonmonogamy).

While my approach to this topic isn't exactly novel, I do believe it is somewhat unique.

Most of the information that you can find online or even in other books approaches the ideals of love and sex through a limited lens, often through things such as Sun sign compatibility or an analysis of Venus and/or Mars, and the nature of sexual expression is usually delineated through the gender binary and an assumption of monogamy. While these approaches might have been more relevant in the past, due in large part to our limited understanding of gender, that is not how I approach sextrology—or astrology in general.

My approach to this topic takes the entire birth chart into account. Just as we are not solely our Sun or Moon or Saturn, neither is our approach to love and sex reflected in just one placement or sign. Relationships, at their core, are just as complex as we are—even more so, perhaps, when you consider that they involve more than just one complicated, beautiful human being. Just as we astrologers interpret the entire chart to gain an understanding of a person's life, we will take the entire chart into consideration when exploring sextrology in this book.

I also don't subscribe to the idea that the planets express themselves differently according to gender or sexuality. A planet may end up playing a more prominent role in one person's chart than it does in another's, but that is based solely on the layout of the chart, which aligns perfectly with who that person is meant to be and nothing more. I also don't use gendered language when talking about astrology. A big reason for this is because the planets exist in all our charts, without exception, regardless of our gender identity or sexuality. A big portion of my background is in linguistics, and I believe that the language we use is important. I also happen to believe that inclusivity is important, and thus I have worked to do away with gendered language in my astrological practice.

The exception to this is when I talk about the feminine and masculine principles where Venus and Mars are concerned. I think it's important to note that these principles have nothing to do with gender, but instead refer to the passive, receptive side of each of us (Venus) and the active side (Mars). This concept is rooted in the larger practices of spirituality and occultism to which I personally subscribe. Whenever these principles and the related language come up in this book, I have done my best to clarify what they mean through the occult lens.

The lens through which I approach sextrology is not about compatibility. It is a focus on the individual at hand—to help each and every one of us to first understand ourselves. Sextrology can help us figure out what we truly desire and what we need to find the fulfillment we are searching for, and identify the types of connections we're looking for to increase our chances of getting what we want. I believe in sexual sovereignty, which is the belief that our sexuality is our own and is not defined by our relationship status, society, or anything else that exists outside of ourselves. In order to truly be empowered when it comes to sex, we need only seek that power within. Once we understand the power that lies within us where sex is concerned, we are then able to share it with others in a way that also feels empowering and find the types of connections we truly desire.

HOW TO USE THIS BOOK

Stellar Sex is designed for self-knowledge and exploration. The goal of this book is to be a comprehensive yet fun reference material that can be easily flipped through to the sections that are relevant to your personal chart. You certainly can read it from cover to cover if you wish, but I recommend reading the sections that relate to your placements first, to initiate your deep dive into sexual empowerment. The book is laid out in easily identifiable sections describing the twelve astrological signs and all the placements contained in a birth chart, respectively. The final portion of this book helps you tie all the information you've learned together in order to form a fluid, tangible whole. My hope is that through learning about the many different parts that make up your sexual and romantic nature, you leave this book feeling empowered with the tools and knowledge you need to start having more fulfilling connections that meet your needs as well as your desires.

The first step in navigating this book is, naturally, to get a copy of your birth chart. In today's world, there are myriad ways to calculate your chart. There are plenty of good free apps and websites available that will populate your chart, including astro.com, astro-seek.com, and the Time Passages app. Just make sure you have the following information handy: your full date of birth, the exact time of your birth (yes, it matters!), and the city of your birth. You may find it useful to write this information down somewhere or have it handy on your phone so you can reference it as you make your way through the contents of this book. It may also be helpful to have a basic understanding of the function of each planet. Again, that information is easily found online for free.

A secondary use of this book is to explore the placements of your loved ones to help you better understand the nature of your connections and how the two (or three or four) of you can come together and nurture your relationship in deeper and more meaningful ways. Understanding their needs, even if solely on an emotional level, can enable greater trust, deeper compassion, and, ideally, more fulfillment on both ends. It can also lead to hotter sex.

Before you depart on your sextrology journey, I would like to say that at the end of the day, nobody is living out your birth chart except you. Just as we are in relationship with each other, the planets in your chart are in relationship with each other too! While much of the information in this book was informed by the real-life experiences of my clients and loved ones, your chart is unique to you, as is your experience in love, romance, sex, relationships, and life as a whole. Due to the unique nature of who you are, astrologically speaking and otherwise, everything you read herein may or may not resonate with you. Take what you find meaningful and leave the rest. Use only what is useful, helpful, and empowering.

ONE LAST THING

Before diving in, here are a few housekeeping items for good measure.

Throughout the book, I will refer to the zodiac signs in terms of their element and modality. For reference, here is an overview of those concepts.

The twelve zodiac signs are divided into four different *elements*—fire, earth, air, and water—with each element containing three signs each:

Fire: Aries, Leo, Sagittarius

Earth: Taurus, Virgo, Capricorn

Air: Gemini, Libra, Aquarius

Water: Cancer, Scorpio, Pisces

The signs are also divided into three *modalities*—cardinal, fixed, and mutable—with each modality containing four signs each:

Cardinal: Aries, Cancer, Libra, Capricorn—The cardinal signs and their respective seasons all begin at the inception of each season. Aries season marks the beginning of spring, Cancer the beginning of summer, and so on. Because of their initiating energies, cardinal signs are the leaders of the zodiac. They possess generative energy and are great at spearheading things and being in charge—which is exactly what they want to be. Even the more understated cardinal signs possess an inherent competence and dominance.

Fixed: Taurus, Leo, Scorpio, Aquarius—The seasons of the fixed signs occur at the height of each season, when we are well into spring, summer, fall, or winter. There is a steadiness to all four of these signs that brings consistency and dependability. The fixed signs are, well, fixed! They are quite stubborn, know exactly what they want and like, and are typically not the type to stray. Because of this, they can become single-minded and/or obsessive, which is not necessarily a bad thing! Their relentless focus makes them capable of accomplishing a great deal.

Mutable: Gemini, Virgo, Sagittarius, Pisces—The mutable signs have their respective moment at the end of each season. As we make our way through the twilight of each season and prepare ourselves for the coming change, the mutable signs aid us in these times of transition and flow. Mutable signs are naturally flexible, adaptable, and open to many perspectives and experiences. They teach us the beauty in going with the flow and being able to see things from different points of view. They know that life is complex and nuanced and many truths can exist at once.

I will also refer to the planets and their respective *dignities*: domicile, exaltation, detriment, and fall. Here is a basic breakdown of what those terms mean:

Domicile: This is the sign (or signs) in which a planet is considered to be at home. It is the sign that the planet rules. In many ways, a planet and its sign of domicile are saying the same thing. A planet in domicile experiences ease of expression and power.

Exaltation: This is a sign whose main characteristics and/or motivations line up well with the nature of the respective planet. Similar to when a planet is in domicile, this is a powerful position for a planet to be in.

Detriment: Signs in detriment are always opposite signs in domicile. For example, Venus is at home (in domicile) in Libra and therefore is in detriment in Aries (since Aries is opposite Libra). Because the nature of the sign is directly opposed to the nature of the planet, many believe that planets in detriment struggle to express themselves the way they want to. While this can be true, it's important not to view this as being negative. Planets in detriment (or fall) can be dynamic and unique and bring something fresh to the table.

Fall: Signs in fall are always opposite signs in exaltation. Again, we see a sharp contrast between the attributes of the sign and the nature of the planet. While the belief is that planets in fall face the same challenge as planets in detriment do, it's not quite as extreme. And, like planets in detriment, planets in fall still have their unique gifts.

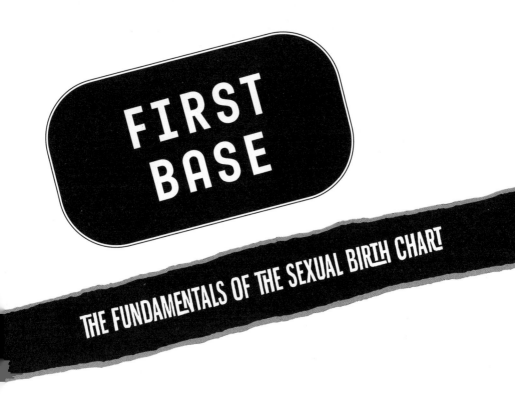

FIRST BASE

THE FUNDAMENTALS OF THE SEXUAL BIRTH CHART

When it comes to unlocking the sexual birth chart, we take the entirety of the chart into account—which is to say we use all the same elements we normally do when doing a normal chart interpretation. However, because we're approaching the chart solely through the lens of sex and love, there are a few changes that must be made before we can understand what we're looking at. In this first section of the book, that's precisely what we'll be doing. And it's true: There are a lot of similarities we'll see between the sexual roles of the planets, points, and houses and the more traditional associations and characteristics you're used to seeing. My hope is that these interpretations will feel pretty intuitive and natural, especially if you're someone who already possesses a basic understanding of astrology.

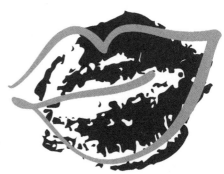

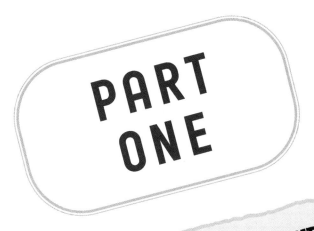

PART ONE

THE PERSONAL PLANETS

In astrology, the personal planets are the planets we feel each and every day of our lives. We experience them on a more tangible level and a more immediate level. The personal planets include the two luminaries (the Sun and the Moon), Mercury, Venus, and Mars. Because of the intimate nature of sextrology, these are the main planets we'll be focusing on in this book, as they are the foundation upon which we are built—and, by extension, the foundation upon which our everyday lives are built. The personal planets make up the very fabric of our erotic selves.

1

THE SUN ☉

DOMICILE: Leo

EXALTATION: Aries

DETRIMENT: Aquarius

FALL: Libra

Where else would we begin our journey except with the Sun, the illustrious ball of life-giving energy that is the center of our solar system and the main luminary in astrology? Sun signs are what we first learn about when we hear about astrology, and they tend to be what is being compared whenever we read about compatibility between signs. And it's true: The Sun plays an all-important role in astrology, as it is our identity, our ego, and the role we're playing out each and every day in our lives. Plus, as the Sun is at home in Leo, a sign that is associated with sex, we would be horribly remiss *not* to include it!

Unlike the typical Sun sign compatibility posts we see online, the role the Sun plays in sextrology points instead to our erogenous identity. It's what we feel and see in our own sexuality and how we show up and embody it.

SUN IN ARIES

We kick off this section, and ultimately this book, with the Sun in the first sign of the zodiac, Aries. The cosmic ram is the first of both the cardinal signs and the fire signs and is where we find the Sun seated in its exaltation.

15

THE SUN POINTS TO OUR EROGENOUS IDENTITY. IT'S WHAT WE FEEL AND SEE IN OUR OWN SEXUALITY AND HOW WE SHOW UP AND EMBODY IT.

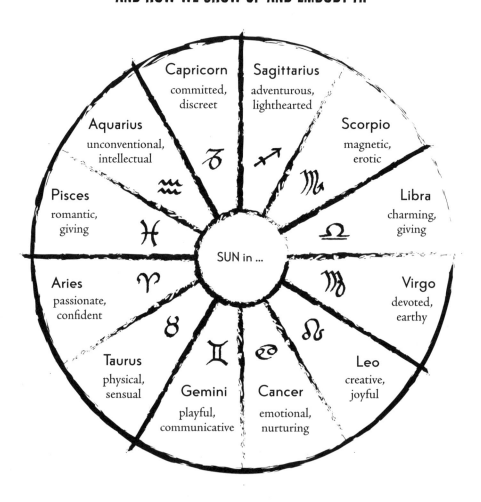

Remember, the status of "exaltation" is given to a sign that shares many of the same qualities, characteristics, and goals as the respective planet—in this case, the Sun. As Aries is the sign of the self, there are obvious connections to identity and individuality, the main components of the Sun. If we had to rank the signs in order of which ones embody their sexuality the most, Aries would come in a close second, neck and neck with the Sun in Leo, the natural champion of this category.

Aries, in general, is fueled by a burning passion within. Thanks to their ruling planet, Mars, these individuals are all about taking action and taking it *now*. As the first of the four cardinal signs, they are initiators. Aries represents the spark of life that emerges from the darkness, the first sprouts that come out of the soil in spring. Indeed, the start of Aries season each year aligns with the vernal equinox, a time when the light begins to take over once again and many, many things begin after lying dormant in winter. This same quality of beginnings is embodied fully within the ram: If you want to get something off the ground, an Aries is the one to call.

Aries individuals are ambitious, driven, and very clear about who they are and what they want. They're also bold as hell and unapologetic about their desires and their individuality. Aries doesn't require the approval of anyone around them, as they know the only true validation they need comes from within. An inherent confidence and courage pulses through the veins of the cosmic ram, making them fantastic leaders and formidable enemies. This is a sign that is unafraid to assert itself and isn't easily intimidated by anyone or anything. These individuals embody the very idea of self-love, and in that sense, they lead by example.

The flip side is that because they're so self-oriented, Aries has a tendency to forget that other people also have wants, needs, and desires. There are plenty of lessons for them to learn around compromise and recognizing the value of the desires and experiences of others in their relationships. However, it's important to note that Aries individuals are extremely loyal to their loved ones and will turn their fierce passion into protecting or standing up for them. In that sense, they make wonderful allies to have on your team.

As far as their relationship to their sexual identity is concerned, the cosmic ram has a natural confidence and ease in this area with their Sun in exaltation. As mentioned earlier, Aries is the sign of the self, and these individuals are very clear about their wants, needs, desires, and who they are, which extends perfectly into the realm of sex, too. Because Aries is ruled by Mars, the planet of sex, the ram exudes a powerful virility and formidable sexual prowess. Aries naturally embodies their passion, possessing a raw and instinctual energy when it comes to their erotic side. Because Aries is the first sign of the zodiac, they also like to keep things fresh in their relationships and lives, striving for a sense of perpetual newness. Aries lives and breathes in the now, having a tendency to get swept up in the heat of the moment. Therefore, it's important for them to be able to cultivate these qualities within their own eroticism, which often translates to a constant need for stimulation, both within themselves and with their partners.

With Aries, we also see a focus on self-love, more than with any other sign, save for Leo. This is a key component for any Aries when it comes to unlocking and embodying their sexuality.

SUN IN TAURUS

In the sign of Taurus, the Sun moves from hot and heavy to cool and sensual. The second sign of the zodiac is the first of the earth signs as well as the first of the fixed signs. The nature of fixed signs is, well, fixed. Each respective season of the fixed signs occurs when we are well into one of the four seasons, and they bring a certain steadfastness to the table—especially, in my opinion, Taurus.

The cosmic bull is nothing if not consistent. Indeed, the hallmark of Taurus can be seen in their desire for not just stability but also predictability. These individuals feel most comfortable in life when they know what's going to happen each day. Taurus loves a good routine and enjoys the mundane and monotonous aspects of life to a degree that we don't see much in the other signs. Thanks to the influence of their ruling planet, Venus, Taurus individuals truly value comfort and ease, hence their desire to create and maintain a life that embodies those qualities.

However, it's important to note that the Taurus desire for predictability also makes these individuals resistant to change. In fact, they can be quite slow in this regard and may even downright fear change. They have a tendency to avoid or delay change as long as possible, often not opting to embrace it until there's pretty much no other choice. Note that Taurus placements can be, well, quite bull-headed! Their stubbornness shines through in lots of avenues, and having to make changes is definitely one of them.

Beyond this, however, Taurus is an extremely hard worker. Though they may be slow to get started, once they do get around to it, they have the stamina and staying power to see it through to the end. They will work as long and hard as they need to in order to get what they want. Their ability to acquire money and resources is what supports their high-end tastes and luxurious lifestyle. Every nice thing they have they've earned.

When thinking about the sexual embodiment of these individuals, Taurus has a healthy drive. As one of the two signs ruled by Venus, their sexual energy manifests in a deeply sensual way, rather than the jackhammer nature we see with Aries. This doesn't make their sex drive any lower, however. As an earth sign, Taurus, too, is quite physical. Remember that sensuality is expressed through all our physical senses: sight, taste, touch, smell, and hearing. The Venusian nature of Taurus creates a desire for gratification and indulgence that can be borderline gluttonous, giving them a bottomless appetite for all pleasures of the flesh. Taurus also loves to take their time and can be quite tactile. Physical touch is huge for these lovers.

Keep in mind, too, that Taurus is the sign of values and resources. For Taurus, empowerment comes through embodying their values around sex. They thrive when they feel resourced through or by their partners as well, which helps them find the safety and stability they so deeply crave. Taurus is rooted deep within the physical and themselves, and consistency is key for them both individually and in relationships.

SUN IN GEMINI

In Gemini, we are initiated into the first of the air signs as well as the mutable signs. Whereas fire signs thrive on action and earth signs thrive on stability, air signs thrive on information. We move into the intellectual realm with Gemini, a sign that is ruled by Mercury, the planet of communication, learning, and travel, where the focus becomes curiosity and exploration. As a mutable sign, Gemini possesses a natural flexibility and adaptability that we see for the first time in the zodiac. Note that all the mutable signs have their respective season in liminal spaces. During Gemini season, we are wrapping up spring in preparation for the beginning of summer.

Gemini is the sign of duality, able to adeptly embody two opposing energies simultaneously, and possesses a changeable nature. Gemini is also extremely cerebral (as are all air signs) and wants to connect with others above all else. In particular, they value a meeting of the minds and an exchange of ideas and perspectives, thanks to all that Mercurial energy. They're also the sign that is the best at putting themselves in other people's shoes: Nobody understands where you're coming from and how/why you have the perspective you do like a Gemini. However, even if this sign understands your feelings, Gemini isn't one for overdone emotions or dramatic displays. They would much rather have an intellectual conversation and analyze the scenario.

Outside of that, Gemini is light and airy and fun! They can be spontaneous and full of adventure, but they can also be quite fickle and change their mind at a moment's notice. They are great initiators but are notoriously awful at actually following through. (Sorry, Gemini!) Their Mercurial minds need a *ton* of stimulation, as they get bored quickly, and before you know it, they'll have already moved on to the next subject (or person!). It can be difficult to keep up with these busy individuals and even harder to keep them engaged.

Above all else, Gemini values open and honest communication. They avidly practice talking through anything and everything—there is no subject off-limits to these individuals. Healthy communication can be hard and is an area most of us need practice in. In that sense, there's much we can learn from anyone with strong Gemini placements.

The embodiment of Gemini's sexual identity shines through their multifaceted nature, too. Variety is the most important thing for this sign, and this extends to their erotic energy as well. They do best when they allow themselves to be fluid and adaptable when it comes to their sexuality. Rigidity and hard boundaries are the kiss of death for Gemini. These individuals need breathing room when it comes to their sexual prowess, allowing their interests and expressions to change, evolve, and come and go at will. They aren't meant to be put in a box. Whereas fixed signs tend to figure out what they like and stick to it time and again, the mutable nature of Gemini demands and commands change. Being able to communicate their nuanced sexual nature will always be the most helpful thing. Gemini individuals change their mind a lot, and that's okay. It enables them to keep things interesting.

SUN IN CANCER

The sign of Cancer is a rather interesting position for the Sun. The cosmic crab is the second of the cardinal signs but the first of the water signs. We leave behind the busyness and intellectual energy of Gemini and plunge deep into the world of emotions. This makes sense when we consider that Cancer is ruled by the Moon, the planet of our emotions.

As a cardinal sign, Cancer initiates us into summertime. Despite all the solar energy present at this time of year, Cancer is actually ruled by the other luminary, the Moon. Thanks to Cancer's ruling planet, which presides over our inner realms and feelings, these individuals are deep, emotional, sensitive, and nurturing. Cancer can be incredibly self-protective, with its hard crabby shell and razor-sharp claws at the ready to protect the soft, squishy body inside. They are also fiercely protective of the ones they love and are deeply intuitive.

In my opinion, it's highly important to remember the cardinal position of Cancer, as these individuals are often reduced to the stereotype of being the crybabies of the zodiac because they're so sensitive. This stereotype has a tendency to eclipse the cardinal qualities of this sign, which is a shame, as Cancer individuals, too, are some of the leaders of astrology. Sensitivity and strength aren't mutually exclusive, and nobody teaches us that more than this sign. It's true that their deeply emotional and nurturing qualities give them a much different style of leadership, but Cancers are some of the most capable folks around. They teach us the value of leading from the heart, from a place of care, and show us the incredible things that can be accomplished when we allow love to be the foundation of all we do.

Beyond this, Cancer is associated with family and the home. Cancers tend to be more introverted and can struggle with a bit of shyness at first, which is ultimately rooted in their need for safety. Unlike Leo, who loves to be the center of attention, Cancer individuals are more likely to take their time and observe, feeling out people, places, and things and discerning whether or not they truly want to open up. They may need to meet you a few times before they start to come out of their shell and feel comfortable.

This idea of safety bleeds over into Cancer's sexual identity. More than for any of the other signs covered so far, emotional intimacy needs to be established first in order for Cancer to truly blossom in their sexual expression. It's extremely important for them to feel safe first within themselves and their physical vessel, as well as within their physical environment, before they will feel empowered enough to allow their sexual energy to come to the surface. Then, of course, there is the Cancer need to feel safe with their partner. Cancers have a need to feel needed, and once they feel this from their partners, that's when they truly thrive.

It's also important for Cancers to experience a bit of playfulness in their sexual expression. So often they get pigeonholed in these matronly, nurturing roles and their playful nature gets forgotten. Allowing room for fun is key for these lovers.

Keep in mind, also, that Cancer rules over the chest and stomach. There's something about showing a little skin in these areas that can help to unlock their eroticism.

SUN IN LEO

At last we arrive in the throne room of the Sun, the seat of its true power, in Leo. The astral lion is the second of both the fire and the fixed signs, with its season occurring during the height of summer. Since Leo is the sign that represents the ego, it makes sense that the Sun is in domicile here. When we speak about the characteristics of Leo and the Sun, we're pretty much saying the same thing twice.

Leos are fun, bold, and creative, with a penchant for drama. They can be larger-than-life in their self-expression, loving to bring a little flair to all they do. They are warmhearted, generous, and charismatic, making them excellent leaders who shine in bringing their unique perspective to all they do. Leos are great problem solvers as well, which enables them to channel their creativity in all kinds of ways and again lends itself to being a visionary leader.

More than any other sign, Leo has a need to stand out from the crowd. They want to be acknowledged for everything that makes them unique, special, and different. These individuals are proud and confident, giving them an incredible amount of personal magnetism. They wish to be seen and appreciated for their strong qualities—which is where their reputation for loving compliments comes in. And it's true: Leos love validation! We all do, of course. Leo just happens to be a little more up-front about it.

Similarly to Cancer, Leo is highly concerned with their inner circle. They want to know the goings-on of their favorite people and will shine their benevolent light on all who are in their favor. As mentioned above, Leo can be extremely generous with those they care about, and this often manifests through them illuminating the unique gifts their loved ones possess. Leo is the ultimate hype man, and they are fiercely loyal to those they love. If ever you're in need of a confidence boost, Leo will dole out the compliments all day long.

Of all the potential positions of the Sun, Leo is the one that embodies their sexuality the most readily and with the most ease. Leo is the sign associated with sex. These individuals possess a natural vitality that lends itself well to sexuality. When their prowess is combined with their innate self-esteem, we see a person who is innately sexually confident. In fact, sex tends to be a big part of a Leo's identity.

Leo individuals are at their best when they are free to be bold and different where their sexuality is concerned. Again, we see their need to stand out and be truly unique, and whenever and however Leo can do this with their erotic nature, they will thrive. Sexual energy is often likened to creative energy, so allowing their creativity to inform their eroticism is key here. It's also important for this sign to have fun with it! Joy, happiness, and play are the pillars of Leo energy, and there's no reason to put those qualities on a shelf here. Joyful self-expression is peak sexual expression for this sign. Even more so than for Aries, self-love is an important matter for Leo.

Beyond that, Leo rules over the back. Exposing the back when dressing or things like back massages can be especially appealing to this sign. Leo also rules over the hair, and taking care of one's luscious locks can up the magnetism as well.

SUN IN VIRGO

The Sun leaves its seat of power behind in Leo when it enters Virgo, the second of both the earth signs and the mutable signs. Interestingly, Virgo is also ruled by Mercury, just like the first mutable sign, Gemini. However, because Virgo is an earth sign, those Mercurial qualities manifest in much different ways than in airy Gemini.

Virgos are sharp, organized, analytical, and ambitious. These individuals are painstakingly detail-oriented and are always armed with a plan. Thanks to their earthy nature, they thrive on logic rather than emotion and are adept at figuring out the best way to get things done. They do have a tendency toward perfectionism, which gives them incredibly high standards for both themselves and other people. In theory, this is fine, but in practice it can morph into the unachievable and manifest as sharp criticism and never feeling like they're good enough. This is a sick joke for Virgos, who, even on their worst days, are usually the most competent people in the room.

Ultimately, Virgo is the sign of devotion and service. Being of service is their love language, as they know that love is truly a verb, and tangible displays that we can see, feel, and grab hold of in some way make love real. Though Virgos may not be prone to the typical displays of romance and affection, there is something arguably more beautiful in showing up in selfless service to those we care about. At the end of the day, Virgo genuinely just wants to help. Their gift for precision and their practical know-how get channeled into trying to help everyone be at their best. They show they care through acts that we can see, hear, touch, and feel, and ultimately they help to make our day-to-day lives easier.

In Virgo we see individuals who are extremely health-conscious, with lives that are built around a solid routine. The Mercurial influence also makes them busy people who are always on the go and have a ton on their plate. Their minds are always turning: The analysis of Virgo never stops, which gives them a keen intelligence and exacting eye. It can also give them some anxiety. It's very important for them to find ways to release perfectionism and solid outlets for their indomitable minds.

In stark contrast to Leo, Virgo has garnered a strange reputation where sex is concerned, as the Virgin of the bunch. It's true that these individuals tend to struggle with their sexuality more than other signs do, but that's simply because their relationship to sex is a bit different from what society tends to portray. This doesn't mean that Virgos aren't just as sexual as the rest of us; it simply means that they have more of a journey around acceptance here than others might.

For Virgos, embodying their erotic energy in an empowering way involves releasing perfectionism and/or the idea that there is a "right" way to do so. There isn't. It's okay to be more reserved, or private, or messy, or however their sexuality wants to express itself. Compassion is actually the most crucial piece of the puzzle here. Virgos need to be able to receive compassion from their partners as well as give it to themselves. Rigidity and overthinking will kill the libido, and being able to get out of their heads will allow for greater ease. Keeping the lights out in the bedroom might help with any apprehension or nervousness and allow them to come into their bodies and into the moment to amp up their enjoyment of sex.

SUN IN LIBRA

In Libra, the golden disc of life finds itself in its fall. As the opposite sign of Aries, Libra is the sign of the other, the sign of partnership, and in many ways represents ideals that are the antithetical to those of the Sun. In this way, we can begin to understand what it means for a planet to be in its fall, when the motivations of the planet seem diametrically opposed to those of the sign—though the disconnect is not quite as extreme as when a planet is in its detriment, which we will see shortly with Sun in Aquarius. In the case of Libra, often referred to as the sign of others, we see this juxtaposition through Libra's association with partnership. Their motivations are fundamentally rooted within other people, a far cry from the self-oriented nature of the Sun.

As the third of the cardinal signs, Libra season begins at the autumnal equinox, when we experience a perfect balance of light and dark in an all-too-poetic initiation. In Libra there exists a true duality where polarity crystallizes in equal measure. Libra understands that light cannot exist without darkness and vice versa; the rectification of anything lies in its opposite. Through giving everything equal and fair weight, true balance is possible.

Libra is the first sign that shifts the focus away from the self and toward others. Libra is ruled by Venus and therefore is highly concerned with relationships. These individuals seek true equality in their partnerships and are quick to stand up against anything that feels unfair or unjust. Under this position of the Sun, our connections with others come forward to take center stage and we begin to learn the value of compromise.

Remember, too, that Libra is a cardinal sign and therefore is one of the leaders of the zodiac. As an air sign, they are sharp and intelligent and know much more than they let on. Thanks to Venus, their ruler, these individuals may hide behind a mask of innocence and charm, making them seem demure and unsuspecting. You can trust, however, that they know exactly what they are doing.

The question of identity takes on a complicated form here, simply because Libras struggle to know themselves outside the context of other people. More than any other sign, Libra experiences other people as a mirror for themselves. This can be both helpful and detrimental, for various reasons. We cannot rely solely on the opinions or reflections of others to define our sense of self. Therefore, Libra can struggle greatly both with codependency and boundaries, as well as needing to find their own autonomy.

As far as sex is concerned, Libra *is* the second sign ruled by Venus, so we do see an affinity here for pleasure, beauty, and indulgence. But whereas the pleasure-focused nature of Taurus is rooted very much in the physical, Libra is rooted in the intellectual realm. Being able to communicate their desires and sexual expression while fostering reciprocity is fundamental for these lovers. Libra's strong need for balance is still present when it comes to sexuality, and others will still act as a mirror here.

Now, when I say this, I don't mean that Libra needs someone else to be able to embody their eroticism. On the contrary, the need to cultivate autonomy is important here as well. But as the sign of partnership, Libra has to learn to prioritize their own wants, needs, and desires just as much as the other person's. In that sense, they will thrive with partners who value Libra's pleasure just as much as their own. In that sense, we see Libra's need to embody their sexuality two ways: both for themselves in general and as a balancing component in their relationships.

Keep in mind that Libra rules over the butt! As of late, the ass has been a big focus in pop culture as far as beauty and sex appeal are concerned. This is Libra's moment to shine, by highlighting their behinds, which can help to unlock their sexual magnetism.

SUN IN SCORPIO

The Sun leaves behind Venus's air temple of Libra and plunges into the deep caverns of Scorpio, the second of both the water signs and the fixed signs. In my opinion, Scorpio is one of the most misunderstood signs out there, which you can see in the way it gets pigeonholed online and in a lot of pop astrology. This probably happens because Scorpio is truly an enigma. Yes, it's a water sign, but traditionally its ruling planet is fiery-ass Mars. People often joke that Scorpio is the fire sign of the water signs, and that might be a good way to think about it. Similar to Aries, its other Mars-ruled counterpart, Scorpio's keyword is *passion*.

Scorpio possesses an unrivaled intensity that boils just beneath the surface at all times. However, this intensity isn't something that is readily shown to others, as Scorpios are notoriously private people. Their symbol, the scorpion, possesses a tough exterior of armor and wields not only dual claws but also a venomous stinger, poised and ready to strike with deadly accuracy should they feel threatened. This is a pretty good analogy for the nature of Scorpio. Their fierce need to protect themselves—similar to Cancer, actually— is because of the sensitive body that lies underneath all that shiny armor.

That's right—Scorpios are some of the deepest feelers in existence, and they're wounded much more easily than they'd ever readily admit to anyone, except for *maybe* a very close few. Their capacity for love runs strong and deep and makes them fierce lovers and friends who are extremely loyal creatures. Note that they typically keep their circles small, as it takes these lovers a long time to trust and open up. They are only willing to share their loyalty and love with those who have been deemed worthy.

As the sign of transformation, Scorpio is constantly engaged in the cycle of life, death, and rebirth, having to embrace change time and again. The superpower of Scorpio lies in their ability to transmute their pain into power, shedding the dead weight in their lives time and again, only to emerge from the ashes of their death cycle more beautiful, powerful, and resplendent than before.

Now, by nature, Scorpios are incredibly sexual creatures. Embodying their powerful erotic energy comes naturally to them—Scorpio rules over the genitals, after all—and they are the only sign that gives Leo a run for their money in this department. The very essence of Scorpio energy expresses itself through animal magnetism. It's dark, sultry, and thick with the promise of deep sexual pleasure, though they'd never say so outright.

Their mysterious energy makes Scorpios incredibly alluring to those around them, and to those with a weaker resolve, they may be downright intimidating. These lovers have incredible personal power, and it radiates from them without them having to say a word.

Thanks to the Martian influence, there is a natural physicality to Scorpio that helps these individuals to be present and grounded within their body, which they have honed to a sharp blade. One thing people often miss about this sign is that they're jocks! Scorpios have a reputation for having a hot body, and it's because they take care of themselves. Just as we see with Aries individuals, their Mars-ruled counterparts, Scorpios have a need to move their body and have an outlet for all their energy. Sex is a great avenue for that, too. Mars gives Scorpio a voracious appetite, and these lovers are ready to devour and burn and pine and perish. Sex can be transformative for them, and their natural, powerful prowess can be transformative for their partners, too.

SUN IN SAGITTARIUS

I find the shift from Scorpio to Sagittarius season to be one of the most palpable ones out there. We leave behind the depths of Scorpio and are immediately flung into the high heavens of Sagittarius, going from one extreme to another. Sagittarius is the final of the three fire signs and the third of the four mutable signs, and it just so happens to be ruled by benevolent Jupiter.

Sagittarius represents the archetypes of the archer, the truth seeker, and the spiritual teacher. There are many cultures that believe enlightenment brings a unique perspective—one from very high up, that enables us to see the master plan, the grand perspective—and with it comes a heavy dose of wisdom. Such is the energy of Sagittarius.

These individuals possess an extreme amount of optimism, faith, and abundance. Thanks to their unbridled trust in the Divine, Sagittarius is able to take life in stride, knowing that everything will work out for them just fine. (Hint: it usually does.) They are here for the adventure we call life, and they know that life is enriched through the vast array of experiences we can have. They'd rather learn how to do something by actually doing it than by reading a book about it. Even though we are moving quickly into the dark and cold of winter during Sagittarius season, this sign brings the light and the warmth to keep us going.

Sagittarians are extremely independent and will not wait around for other people. They are on a mission to go do what they want to do, and if you aren't ready to join them at a moment's notice, you'll get left in the dust! Because of their big-picture approach to things, these lovers tend to stay unbothered by most things. They know there's no point in sweating the small stuff, and they don't have time to get twisted up in other people's drama. They've got a flight to catch, after all.

Thanks to Jupiter, their ruling planet, Sagittarians do spend a lot of time thinking about what it all means. They are constantly trying to figure out what they believe in that's higher or bigger than themselves and are concerned with the grander questions about life. Certainly they love to share their beliefs with others, are down for deeply philosophical discussions, revel in a good debate, and love, love, love to laugh.

The erotic nature of a Sagittarius expresses itself most readily through humor, in fact. These individuals love to poke and prod and tease, and love it when somebody can make them laugh right back. There's something about witty banter that really revs them up.

More than any other sign in the zodiac, Sagittarius lovers are sexual intellectuals. Similar to what we see in their opposite sign, Gemini, Sagittarians love to connect with others in the intellectual sphere, and the key is to engage their mind before anything else. Eroticism is unlocked for them via the mind.

The erotic nature of Sagittarius is actually quite lighthearted. Because it's a fire sign, certainly there's a healthy sex drive here, and Sagittarians bring their adventurous spirit to the bedroom. That's right—just like everything else they're interested in, sex needs to be an avenue to expansion and growth, and this manifests as a fun, lively approach to sex and a lover who is down to try it all. Again we see the Sagittarius desire to learn through firsthand experience, and what better way to do that than through many different lovers and ways and places to fuck?

Because of both Sagittarius's and Jupiter's connection to faraway lands and different cultures, we may also see someone who is attracted to accents and people from different cultural backgrounds.

SUN IN CAPRICORN

When the Sun moves from Sagittarius into Capricorn, we are again greeted with a tangible shift in energy. We are pulled from the skies back down to planet Earth and therefore back to reality. Capricorn is the final of the three cardinal signs, and the final of the four earth signs, too, but it's the first of the two signs ruled by heavy-hitting Saturn. (Saturn is the traditional ruler of Aquarius.) As with the rest of the cardinal signs, Capricorn initiates us into a new season—winter—and begins on the winter solstice each year.

Somehow, over time, Capricorns have been pigeonholed into being thought of as obsessed with money, power, their career, and little else. While Capricorns *are* quite ambitious and tend to channel that ambition into their careers, to say that's all they're about is a horrible disservice to the cosmic sea goat.

As the opposite sign of Cancer, Capricorn makes up the other end of the nurturing axis in astrology. As an earth sign, Capricorn's approach to nurturing is much more practical. They are focused on things that are tangible, that can be checked off a list, such as paying the bills. But they, too, are focused on taking care of their loved ones. They just do it through avenues that create stability, and they are realistic enough to understand that just existing in the world requires money and therefore a job to supply it. Capricorn *is* the first Saturn-ruled sign (traditionally) and therefore manifests its qualities of structure, stability, and working hard toward something over the long term in order to achieve a bigger payoff.

Capricorns also possess a great deal of wisdom. Thanks to the maturity Saturn bestows upon them, they value responsibility and integrity, and because of this they likely had to grow up pretty fast for one reason or another. Their life experience has therefore granted these lovers a deep well of knowledge and maturity. They are wonderful people to turn to for advice.

This wisdom also manifests in a well-developed intuition. I think people often forget the sea aspect of the sea goat. Yes, Capricorn is an earth sign, but again, through their maturity and experience they have also learned the value of listening to their instincts and that inner voice. They know when it's time to be practical and when it's time to let their intuition speak and guide them.

For those with the Sun in Capricorn, their sexual identity is rooted in societal ideals and traditional norms—namely, the ones they were raised with. This identity is a blend of whatever values were instilled in them growing up, as well as whatever messages they've received and ideas they've been indoctrinated into via society and culture. Now, this isn't to say these individuals can't think for themselves. Of course they can, but because Capricorn represents society, authority, and traditional values, it's not shocking to see these play out through the sexual lens either. That said, there's usually a journey for Caps around having to dismantle outdated ideals and breaking free from the chains of expectations from said society, family, etc., which includes sex.

It's true that Capricorns are a bit more reserved when it comes to sex—at least on the outside. They're not the type to kiss and tell or speak about their sexual escapades, as it's not a topic of polite conversation. Don't let their reserved nature fool you, though, as they're probably having a lot of sex! Capricorns love to be in charge, and this extends to the bedroom. Though they won't sleep with just anybody, Capricorns have a healthy sex drive and will go after who they want directly, just like everything else in life. They are dominant, steady, and long-lasting, if you know what I mean.

The foundation of Capricorn's erotic nature is truly built upon integrity. Where values and being a good person are concerned, Capricorn is the sign that leads by example when it comes to actually walking the walk, and this admirable quality gets channeled into their approach to love, sex, and partnerships. Capricorns hold themselves to a high standard and are unlikely to compromise those standards or be dishonest about who they are and what they want and stand for.

SUN IN AQUARIUS

In the second-to-last sign of the zodiac, we see the Sun in its only sign of detriment, Aquarius. The water bearer is ultimately about community: Aquarius is focused on humanitarian issues and strives for the greater good of all, not just the self. This lack of a self-focused nature, therefore, has the Sun—the very manifestation of the self—struggling to carry out its mission. However, there is a curious dichotomy that exists within Aquarius. Yes, they want to see the highest good of humanity come to fruition, but they also pretty much want to be left to their own devices. Make no mistake—just because the Sun is in detriment here doesn't mean that Aquarius has no sense of self. On the contrary, Aquarians are some of the most unique individuals around!

Aquarius wants nothing more than the freedom to live their life the way they want to and be free to be who they are, whether other people understand it or not. In fact, we can see the stubborn nature of this fixed air sign whenever somebody tries to tell them what not to be or feel or think or do. Suddenly these normally agreeable folks will transform into a brick wall and not only will keep doing what they were doing but will amp it up even more simply to spite you!

Because the very nature of Aquarius points to the fringes and being different from everyone else, these creatures often feel alienated and can spend their lives feeling misunderstood, like they're on the outside looking in. It's actually quite important for these folks to find their group, likely a mixed bag of friends, family, and lovers who truly see them, understand them, and radically accept them for who they are.

Now, when we consider how Aquarians approach their sexual identity, this is, naturally, quite different, too. On the one hand, we can see individuals who harbor unconventional ideals when it comes to love and sex. In fact, their erotic philosophies may go directly against what society at large tends to value or expect in that department. In that sense, they can be pretty kinky and open to all kinds of things, including engaging in different kinds of relationships besides monogamy. This isn't always true, however. Because the very nature of Aquarius is unexpected, the erotic nature of these lovers, more than any other sign, can manifest any which way and certainly can't be put in a box. Because of their subversive approach to sex and love, Aquarius lovers pave the way for the rest of us when it comes to advancing or evolving our ideals as a society. They are waymakers in all they do, and sex is no exception. One thing you can count on, though, is that Aquarians will always be attracted to strong individuals just like them. These lovers are the best at seeing and appreciating the quirks and unique characteristics in others that may often be overlooked, and truly that is what attracts them the most.

However, in stark contrast to their opposite sign, Leo, which rules over sex, Aquarius is the sign that tends to like the *idea* of sex rather than actually having it. In fact, they may feel more aroused when their partner(s) are unavailable in some way or are acting aloof—which is to say they experience desire for their partners the most when they aren't around. This can be maddening for their partners, of course, but Aquarius needs space, and it is in this space that their desire has room to blossom. Keep in mind that Aquarius *is* a fixed sign, and once these lovers have found someone they are truly interested in, they're going to do what fixed signs do best: fixate.

A foundation of friendship in a relationship is crucial for Aquarians. This is where the classic friends-to-lovers archetype comes to life, as it's important that they genuinely like their partners, not just love them.

SUN IN PISCES

We end the zodiacal journey with Pisces, the last of the water signs as well as the mutable signs. Pisces season carries us through the end of winter, preparing us for the astrological New Year with the blooming of spring. In the final astrological sign, we see the Sun continuing to build upon the humanitarian themes of Aquarius and expanding them out even further. Of all twelve signs, Pisces is the most spiritual. There's something about the individuals that seems to exist in another dimension entirely, as they possess a powerful intuition that makes them borderline or even downright psychic.

Because they are so tapped into the ethereal channels of existence, Pisces are able to sense and understand the way those around them are feeling. The Pisces capacity for empathy, love, compassion, and understanding is unmatched. They embody the ideal of unconditional love in a way the rest of us don't and honestly probably can't. This quality makes them excellent healers, mystics, counselors, and the like. As the opposite sign of Virgo, Pisces is the other sign of service and tends to be self-sacrificing in the name of love and humanity. While this is a beautiful and important quality to have, these lovers have to be especially careful about and aware of boundaries. It's too easy for them to be taken advantage of by those who don't share the same kind heart. Just because they can see the beauty in others doesn't mean everyone else can do the same. The porous nature of Pisces can make it difficult for these lovers to establish boundaries, especially because this may seem to go directly against their empathetic nature. At some point in their lives, there's usually a hard lesson or two that ends up teaching them the value of having said boundaries.

The ethereal nature of Pisces also manifests through a powerful imagination and creativity. Very often these lovers are artists, poets, visionaries, and dreamers. They are the true romantics of the zodiac and are here to bring their rose-colored visions to life. Their soft hearts are open and perpetually in bloom, paving the way for the rest of us. Truly Pisces leads by example when it comes to the idealistic version of humanity, never allowing the harshness of reality to harden their hearts.

One thing to keep in mind, however, is that Pisces's strong aversion to the harshness of reality often manifests through a need to escape. We all engage in escapism somehow, but none of us do it quite like Pisces. The actual escape route can show up in any number of ways: drugs, sex, video games, TV, art, writing, whatever. It's just important that this means of escape doesn't turn into self-destruction or completely inhibit their ability to see and live in reality. Sometimes the fantasy of Pisces can turn sour and morph into delusion. Learning how to ground themselves and find healthy means of escape and coping mechanisms is a must!

Now, the sexual identity of Pisces is highly fluid. Because of their mutable nature, their erotic energies are constantly ebbing and flowing, as changeable as the tides. And that's okay. In fact, trying to box themselves into one thing or another or having any rigidity whatsoever around their sexuality will only stifle them. Pisces lovers are forever looking to please their partners. They are givers in the bedroom and stay ready to mold and shape themselves accordingly. This, too, will influence the way their eroticism manifests and again will reinforce the changeability of it all.

However, at one point or another, it's important for these lovers to be in touch with their sexuality outside the context of their partner(s). Sex doesn't have to equal sacrifice, and learning to own their wants, needs, and desires is so important. Pisces naturally embodies a fantastical, dreamy aura, and I promise they have fantasies of their own. Learning to speak up and ask for those things in the bedroom is key. Certainly they could benefit from having partners who are givers in the bedroom, too. But in the end, embracing the natural cycles of their erotic nature is the best thing they can do for themselves.

A NOTE ON THE HOUSES

In the birth chart, the house the Sun lives in points to the area of our lives that much of our energy, self-esteem, and (sexual) identity is tied up in. For example, someone with their Sun in the sixth house may spend a lot of time and energy focusing on their health and/or job. For someone with their Sun in the seventh house, much of their identity and sense of self-worth may be dependent upon their current relationship status.

The house of the Sun can point to where we naturally shine in terms of our unique gifts and talents, too, or where we desire attention and validation. This desire for validation can also be seen through the lens of sextrology. Someone with their Sun in the tenth house may enjoy a lot of sexual attention or be seen as a person who is attractive and desirable, for example, whereas someone with their Sun in the fourth house is likely to be much more private and may feel uncomfortable or downright unsafe receiving overt sexual attention from others. Make sure to read up on the house your Sun sits in later in this book (chapter 17) for further understanding.

As a final note, the Sun, the first luminary in the chart, finds its joy in the ninth house. Planetary joys are a concept rooted in Hellenistic (which is to say traditional) astrology and point to an area in the chart where a planet is said to be, well, joyful. This is a place of ease and power for that planet, where it operates well. Note that because this is a practice rooted in a time when only the seven traditional planets were known, this concept doesn't extend to the modern planets, Uranus, Neptune, and Pluto.

The concept of planetary joys points to certain houses in the chart where planets find an ease of expression. The ninth house is the house of joy for the Sun. Hellenistic astrology refers to this house as the "place of God," and as the Sun has deep roots in religion and spirituality as a literal representation of God, this connection makes sense. Those with their Sun in the ninth house are optimistic and joyful and have an incredible faith in something higher than themselves. They may be religious, mystical, spiritual, and/or philosophical. Certainly there is an interest in travel, education, and a pursuit to find the truth of all things. These lovers are often interested in other cultures and may speak a foreign language or two. They may even be attracted to people who have an accent and are from another country or at least have a different cultural background.

People with their Sun in the ninth house have concerns that lie within the bigger picture of life, searching to find the role they play and how they fit into the world at large. Their beliefs and ethics are of great importance, and they may even wish to impart their wisdom and knowledge to others. They likely spend a lot of time thinking about the bigger questions in life and are certainly looking for someone who wants to discuss such matters and strike out into the world to experience and learn as much as they can together. There is an undeniable zest for the width and breadth and depth of life, which they are looking to experience as much as is humanly possible.

2

THE MOON ☾

DOMICILE: Cancer
EXALTATION: Taurus
DETRIMENT: Capricorn
FALL: Scorpio

As the second luminary in the birth chart, the Moon plays an all-important role in our experience of relationships. This is the first section where we'll depart from looking at a planet and its relationship to sex in an overt manner and shift more toward the other components that make up our relationships. The Moon deals mainly with our emotions, but that doesn't mean there isn't a connection to our erotic selves. Indeed, for many, and to some extent, I would argue, for all of us, the emotional connection will eventually come into play in the bedroom. Even the most casually oriented of us will eventually find ourselves in a serious relationship or with some serious feelings for someone. With that, I invite you to consider the following and how it shows up for you where sex is concerned

The Moon rules over our complex inner realms. It's our emotions, our intuition, the way we take in and process things. It points to our definition of nurturing and what we need to feel safe and secure within relationships. It also rules over our physical body traditionally and can point to what we need to feel not only safe in our home and immediate environment but also safe and nurtured within our physical vessel. The Moon also rules over the subconscious, where our deepest desires and wounds tend to hide.

39

THE MOON POINTS TO OUR DEFINITION OF NURTURING AND WHAT WE NEED TO FEEL SAFE AND SECURE IN RELATIONSHIPS. IT'S OUR EMOTIONS AND OUR INTUITION.

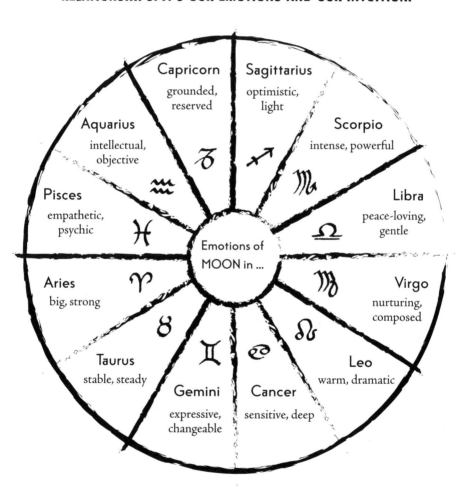

Emotions of MOON in ...

Capricorn grounded, reserved

Sagittarius optimistic, light

Aquarius intellectual, objective

Scorpio intense, powerful

Pisces empathetic, psychic

Libra peace-loving, gentle

Aries big, strong

Virgo nurturing, composed

Taurus stable, steady

Leo warm, dramatic

Gemini expressive, changeable

Cancer sensitive, deep

Safety is an incredibly important component within relationships. This is something that I tout relentlessly to my clients and that I feel is often overlooked when thinking about relationships. Not all of us were raised in a safe environment, and unfortunately interpersonal violence is all too common in romantic relationships. Experiencing these traumas deeply shifts our relationship to our own bodies and environments, not to mention our relationships to other people. If we cannot feel safe (emotionally, mentally, physically, and spiritually) with someone else, we are setting ourselves and the connection up for failure. When it comes to sexual exploration and experimentation, safety is incredibly important as well.

MOON IN ARIES

The Moon in Aries has *big* feelings. They aren't happy; they're elated. They aren't sad; they're devastated. They aren't angry; they're livid. You get the idea.

Aries stokes the fire on any and all emotions, elevating them to enormous heights, so they tend to rise quickly and take on a larger-than-life form. Truly these people have no chill. Because of this, a Lunar Aries has a sense of urgency around their emotions. Everything can feel like an emergency that needs to be addressed and remedied *right now*. This urgency can be frustrating both for the Aries Moon person and the people around them, especially because the intensity of those emotions can feel all-consuming and eclipse the feelings of anyone else, and then once those feelings have been voiced, they leave just as quickly as they arrived.

This dynamic tends to be stronger when a person with an Aries Moon is younger, though there are plenty of real-life factors and choices on their part that can influence how true that is. There are lots of lessons for them around learning to consider the feelings of other people and recognizing that they aren't the only one who has feelings, needs, etc. Learning to consider other people in general can be a big lesson for any Aries placement, as the sign of the self has to learn about its counterpart, the other.

At the end of the day, an Aries Moon needs their feelings to be heard and validated. While this is true for everyone, the Aries Moon has an arguably stronger, more up-front need for this than the other positions of the

Moon. It's also important that their loved ones don't try to shame them for the passion that runs through their feelings or give them messages of being "too much." Aries feels a strong need to voice their thoughts and feelings and will do best in relationships where those feelings are heard and valued. Keep in mind that Aries is fiercely loyal and will defend their people unwaveringly. Thus, whenever a Lunar Aries feels valued, they will value others in kind.

MOON IN TAURUS

The Moon is exalted in Taurus, meaning there is a cohesiveness between the characteristics of the cosmic bull and the qualities of the Moon. In short, the Moon feels good in the second sign of the zodiac.

In my opinion, this is where we first see the themes of the home that the Moon points to. There is nothing a Taurus loves more than their personal space. They devote much time and energy to cultivating an oasis of comfort full of earthly, sensual pleasures. Thanks to their Venusian nature, Taurus wants their place to look good, feel good, smell good, and taste good. You'll know you're in the home of a Taurus when you smell incense or candles burning, eat yummy food, and sit on a couch full of lush pillows and blankets. While their aesthetic preferences are, of course, subjective, a Lunar Taurus absolutely loves to decorate and curate according to their preferences. These people tend to be much more introverted and spend a lot of time at home, so it's important that their space is a place where they actually want to be.

Unlike Aries, a Taurus Moon tends to be pretty chill. As with all earth sign Moons, there is an even keel to the emotions, a groundedness that lends itself first to practicality. Because of this, a Taurus Moon is pretty stable in their approach to emotions. They possess a steadiness that makes them slow to express grand displays of emotion. In fact, a Taurus Moon loves to take their time with pretty much everything in general, including reacting and opening up emotionally.

However, like all Taurus placements, there is an inherent stubborn streak that runs through this position of the Moon. Generally speaking, Taurus doesn't like being told what to do. Through the lunar lens, this manifests as being told how they feel, what they feel, or what they should or shouldn't be feeling. Trying to control a Taurus or push them to change will only result in them digging their heels deeper into the earth while they keep right on doing that thing. It's best to let them have their process and work through their emotions at their own pace, even if it does feel maddeningly slow.

Above all else, a Taurus Moon needs consistency. More than any other sign, Taurus thrives on predictability. They love their routines and feel best when they know what to expect. This desire extends to their relationships, and their most fulfilling connections come through people they know they can depend on.

MOON IN GEMINI

With the Moon in the air temple of Gemini, we see someone who has variable emotions. Gemini is a mutable sign, and because of this, their feelings change quickly. They can go from one extreme to the other within a matter of moments and can run the entire spectrum of emotions in a matter of days or even hours.

Part of this is due to the duality of this sign. Since Gemini is the sign of the twins, we look at the idea of self versus other, and a Gemini Moon is quick to observe and take in the environment around them. They may often have to discern whether what they're feeling is truly their emotion or if they've taken on that feeling because it's what someone around them is experiencing. Their gut reaction may not entirely be their own, and it is always helpful for them to take a step back and check in with themselves. And, yes, a Gemini Moon wants to talk about their feelings—remember, they have that Mercurial influence!

Typically when it comes to air Moons, we see a person who has a tendency to intellectualize their feelings instead of actually *feeling* them. However, of the three air signs, Gemini is the most likely to be in touch with their emotions and wants to connect with others. If Gemini is going to talk to one person about their feelings, they're going to talk to three or four. Again we see the dualistic nature of this sign come into play through needing other people to act as a mirror, enabling the Gemini Moon to work through their feelings and discern what is truly going on. Keep in mind that meeting the needs of a

Gemini Moon involves active listening. They need to know they've truly been heard and they're actually looking to hear your point of view on the matter. A Lunar Gemini can truly benefit from listening to different points of view or even having their feelings challenged. One of the gifts of Gemini is being able to see things from myriad perspectives, and viewing their feelings through a different lens can be truly beneficial for them.

Thanks to their chatty, social disposition, Gemini Moons also love to get to know the people around them. This group loves to get to know their neighbors, the barista serving them coffee, or whoever they interact with a lot in their local environment.

MOON IN CANCER

The second luminary finds its only home in Cancer, the cardinal water sign of the zodiac. This is an especially strong placement of the Moon. In Cancer, the Moon is deeply intuitive, with a focus on themes of nurturing, safety, family, and tradition.

Moon in Cancer individuals are sensitive and empathetic. They are highly attuned to both their own emotions and those of others, often experiencing a strong emotional response to the world around them. People with this position of the Moon can be, well, moody. Just as the Moon moves through its phases, so, too, can their feelings fluctuate greatly. These lovers need a fair amount of alone time to be able to wade through all their deep emotions.

As Cancer is the sign of the mother and the home, these lunar lovers often have a strong nurturing instinct, gaining the reputation of being the moms (or whichever parent was more nurturing) of the zodiac. They feel a deep sense of responsibility for their loved ones and may go to great lengths to provide comfort and support. It's important for their partners to keep in mind that these lovers need support and care as well. Too often those with Cancer placements end up being the giver and forget that they need to receive (and deserve to receive) just as much. In my opinion, this is especially important for Cancer Moons, as the Moon is all about receiving.

Inevitably, a Lunar Cancer will be somewhat of a homebody, even if they have other placements that tend to be more outgoing and social. As a rule,

Cancers love to be at home. It's where they feel the most comfortable and safe, and they spend much energy turning their personal space into a warm, inviting oasis. They love their home partly because that's where the family is! Family is very important to Cancer, and especially with the Moon here, these lovers are family-oriented, valuing their own family and likely wanting to have one of their own someday. They make wonderful, caring parents and pride themselves on being able to provide loving care.

Safety comes first for a Cancer Moon in order to get their emotional needs met. Because of their self-protective instincts, these lovers may come off as a bit shy or reserved at first. These are the people who need time to observe. They will take time opening up and may need to meet someone a few times or hang back at social events in order to feel people out and decide if it's safe for them to open up and share. In that sense, they need people who are patient and understanding and won't try to force them to open up before they're ready.

Once that trust has been established, their needs lie almost solely in the emotional realm. A Cancer Moon needs someone who values their feelings, will validate their experiences, and will meet them with as much care and kindness as they show. Having a partner who shares the same values, commitment, and long-term goals will keep their appetite fed and help them to experience the fulfillment they seek.

MOON IN LEO

The Moon in Leo actually shares some qualities with the Moon in Cancer. They, too, are highly concerned with their innermost circle, which is often a blend of family, friends, and lovers. Leo absolutely loves to know what's going on in the lives of their people, and especially where the Moon in this sign is concerned, they will expend much of their generosity and organizational skills on these close connections, seeking to help them where they can. As a fixed sign, however, they have to watch out for their need to control bleeding over into trying to control the lives of their inner circle, even if their heart is in the right place.

Indeed, the warmhearted nature of the lion shines through the lens of the Moon. They have lots of love to give and have no qualms about dishing it out in heaps and heaps. As with any Leo placement, a Leo Moon is someone who is supportive and friendly and will always work to lift up those around them. The natural magnetism of this sign lies in their charisma and warmth, and Lunar Leos attract others to them through these qualities.

Certainly these lovers are very proud, if not a bit bossy. Once their pride has been hurt, they can be prone to the typical dramatic behavior that Leo is known for: huffing and puffing and putting on a big show of emotion or complaining or sulking loudly. However, it's likely they'll only do this in the privacy of their home or behind closed doors, as a Leo Moon lover wouldn't be caught dead putting on such a show in public. Their pride keeps them highly concerned about appearances, and they wouldn't do anything that would potentially tarnish their reputation. However, when they're upset, it can be especially difficult to change their mind, which is the hallmark of all the fixed signs. Once the big emotional displays have passed, they are much easier to reason with. Be prepared to apologize first, though!

Getting their emotional needs met is a big deal for these lion lovers. It's important to keep in mind that for as much love as a Leo Moon dishes out, they need just as much love and care in return. Without a healthy amount of it, they can struggle to function in the world. They therefore need a partner who is just as open, warm, and generous with their love and will give it back freely. Leo Moons need to be appreciated for all the attention and intention they put into their relationships, and they thrive on compliments just as much as any other Leo placement. Through the lens of the Moon, the Leo need for attention and validation might be even stronger than for a Leo Sun, and that's okay. Owning the need to be acknowledged and appreciated for all their gifts and talents, rather than feeling embarrassed about it, will actually set these lovers free.

MOON IN VIRGO

In earthy Virgo, the Moon takes on a highly practical energy. More than with any other position of the Moon, we see someone who is concerned with the ins and outs of everyday life. Virgo Moons stay busy tending to all the details and tasks that life demands, taking care of absolutely everything. In fact, being able to attend to things like chores, paying bills, and running errands keeps these lovers perfectly content, feeling safe and secure. As boring as it may sound to other people—or simply those without any Virgo in their chart—Lunar Virgo babes couldn't be happier living a regular, unassuming life.

As with all Virgo placements, the Moon in Virgo seeks to nurture others. Acts of service is how these lunar lovers show they care. They have a strong need to feel useful, as they are, in fact, the *sign* of service, and in that sense they have a strong need to help. And as long as they're appreciated for all the small things they do each day, a Virgo Moon will take care of your life, too.

As a rule, Virgo appreciates efficiency, which often translates into simplicity. They love to streamline processes as much as possible and aren't ones for anything too showy or grandiose. In this way they are the complete opposite of Leo, for example, and will wither under too much overt attention. Lunar Virgos are much more reserved, especially with their feelings, and because of this they may come off as a bit shy or lacking in confidence.

However, I would argue most of the time that probably isn't true. As an earth sign, Virgo isn't a particularly emotional placement of the Moon. These lovers tend to be much more logical and are highly analytical with their feelings. They are more likely to intellectualize and work through their feelings than to engage in some grand display of emotion one way or another. And though they may not be super emotional, they are certainly willing to talk things out.

Virgo Moons get their needs met through having a healthy life. They thrive on routine, structure, and taking care of their physical vessel. Traditionally the Moon represents the body in astrology, and we see that association shine through the most here. Having a partner who values their own health is the best thing for a Virgo Moon, and as low-maintenance as they may be in a lot of ways, having someone who is going to help make their lives easier instead of adding more to their plate is key. They also need someone who is reliable, follows through on their words, and sticks to the plan. These lovers can struggle with anxiety and don't tend to fare well when something isn't going according to plan, so having someone who understands these things about them and will work to neutralize their anxiety will be deeply fulfilling for them.

MOON IN LIBRA

Of all the air signs, the Moon in Libra is surprisingly sensitive. Often referred to as the water sign of the air signs within astrology circles, Libra's sensitive energy is most obvious through the lunar lens.

More than any other position of the Moon, these lovers are highly focused on partnership, as is the Libran way. In fact, they are at their best when they are in a relationship, finding strength, confidence, safety, and security through someone else. This isn't to say they aren't capable of being on their own, but having someone to process their feelings and do life with checks their boxes in a way nothing else quite does. (I would know.)

As with all Libra placements, we see a need for peace, tranquility, harmony, and equality. In the case of the Moon in Libra, we see a striving for these things rather than an inherent existence of them. In fact, these lovers can be quite nitpicky and perfectionistic in their pursuit of harmony and peace, seeming to always find something that needs to be improved or changed. While you may think this is more of a Virgo quality, through the lens of the Moon this actually shows up in Libra, whereas Virgo Moons are much easier to please. In a sick twist of irony, the constant complaining of a Libra Moon can actually stir up a lot of tension with their loved ones, causing much discontent in their relationships. However, because of their desire for peace, these lovers are apt to compromise and concede, especially with acquaintances, although with their long-term partners they are more likely to argue until they win.

That said, the nature of a Lunar Libra is to be highly concerned with others. They are empathetic and understanding, with a focus on the wants, needs, and feelings of those they're close to. These lovers are gentle, sensitive, and charming, possessing the grace of Venus, which they channel into their homes and relationships.

Beyond simply being partnered up, Lunar Libras get their needs met through true equality in relationships. Because their default will always be to prioritize and focus on others, they need people around them who are going to prioritize and value them in return. An even give-and-take in their relationships is crucial. These lovers have to learn that their feelings matter just as much as other people's. In that sense, boundaries are important, too. Moon in Libra lovers can struggle with codependency more than any other Libra placement, and having healthy boundaries in place helps them to gain and maintain a sense of autonomy and the self-confidence that comes with it.

MOON IN SCORPIO

In psychic Scorpio, the Moon is said to be in its fall, which is kind of interesting considering the astral scorpion is a water sign and, just like Cancer and Pisces, is full of deep emotions. In fact, this is easily the most intense position of the Moon, and these lovers actively seek out the emotional intensity they possess in their connections with others. Thanks to the psychic nature of Scorpio being amplified by the Moon, these lovers have a piercing perception that can easily cut through the fluff and enables them to see straight through to the heart of a person or situation. This supernatural ability is sensed by those around them, which can give Scorpio Moons an intimidating aura that either draws people in or repels them. Scorpios operate in extremes, and people either love or hate them.

The deep feeling nature of Scorpio is amplified under the lunar influence, and most people with this placement have a powerful emotional life. Many Scorpio Moons struggle greatly with their intense emotions, which they often feel are outside of their control. They can experience great emotional upheaval in their lives through deeply painful experiences that can bring dramatic ups and downs but ultimately act as catalysts for change and transformation. Remember that Scorpios have an insane amount of emotional fortitude, and they will use that strength to transmute pain into power.

Similar to what we see with Venus in Scorpio, Lunar Scorpio lovers seek out all-consuming relationships and won't waste their time on anything vapid or casual. They find no meaning in surface-level connections and therefore often have a small inner circle of people they're close with. Their private and suspicious nature makes it difficult for them to trust others and feel safe enough to open up and share, so once someone has earned their trust, a Scorpio Moon is going to keep them close. These lovers also don't do anything by halves. They will settle for nothing less than the deepest emotional intimacy possible, so you're either all the way in or all the way out.

For these lovers, getting their emotional needs met involves embracing their desire for intense experiences and relationships. Oftentimes Scorpio Moons try to talk themselves out of their own natural energy because they struggle to find others who share that same desire and can meet them blow for blow in the intensity department. However, it's crucial that these lovers learn to accept their need for intensity and focus on having relationships with people who share that same depth. Frankly, they'd never be satisfied with anything less, so what's the point in settling?

Once a Scorpio Moon can accept that having powerful and transformative emotional experiences is a true need, the upheaval in their life stops being so dramatic.

MOON IN SAGITTARIUS

The Moon in Sagittarius is a fun one. These lunar babes are chock-full of optimism, humor, and a fiery streak. Their jovial nature manifests through viewing life as one big party, with life innately possessing a hint of exoticism and potential. They have a strong need for independence and freedom, and as long as these lovers can get the space they need, they're happy, easygoing folks.

One thing to note about those with their Moon in Sagittarius is that they get bored easily. They need a lot of activity and stimulation in their lives in order to feel satisfied, and therefore they're quite social creatures. These individuals love to go out and meet new people, have new experiences, and travel, travel, travel, travel. As with all Sagittarius placements, they crave adventure and want to experience all that life has to offer, so striking out into the world to explore, ask questions, and learn is highly important to a Sag Moon. Even their homes are often bright, open spaces.

The flip side of this, however, is that because they're always on the go, they can be a bit unorganized. Lunar Sagittarians may struggle to remember appointments and obligations and will probably be late or may not even show up at all! While this can obviously cause issues, it's pretty hard to remain cross with a Sag Moon, as they're too cheerful and hilarious to ignore. Plus, their heart is usually in the right place, even if they aren't physically in the right place. However, at the core of it all, these lovers want nothing to do with a rigid routine or ordinary life that others may lead, as that does nothing except stifle their freedom.

The quintessential faith in the Divine that Sagittarius is known for shows up through the lens of the Moon, too. These lovers believe that everything will just work out for them, and most of the time it does. The inherently spiritual nature of the cosmic archer shines through the Moon, as the themes of both marry well in that sense. Their spiritual wisdom and intuitive nature are strong, and they readily trust in the unfolding of their path.

When thinking about what these lovers need to feel nurtured, they're pretty low-maintenance. This isn't to say that Sagittarius Moons *don't* have emotional needs, but they're so independent that all they truly require from others is space and someone to share all their philosophical musings with. These babes prefer to keep things light and will actually flee from connections that are too intense or overdone. They really aren't ones for grand displays of emotion and much prefer having relationships with others who share their sense of adventure and are down to ride. Truly, the best thing you can do for a Sag Moon is book a flight and go see the world with them.

MOON IN CAPRICORN

As the opposite sign of Cancer, Capricorn is where the Moon is said to be in detriment, struggling to embody all its emotional, nurturing sensibilities in this reserved, practical sign.

More than in any other sign, the Moon in Capricorn is extremely reserved with their emotions. In a way, this can come across quite similar to a Scorpio Moon as far as privacy is concerned, but we don't see the same emotional intensity, thanks to Capricorn being an earth sign.

Just like their other earthy counterparts, Lunar Capricorns are grounded where feelings are concerned, giving them an impressive stability in their disposition. A Capricorn Moon feels like a towering mountain: immovable, unwavering, and eternal. These lovers know how to stay calm in the face of adversity and are quick to prioritize a logical response over any kind of emotionally charged reaction. The term "cool, calm, and collected" was coined for these babes!

However, it's important to keep in mind the Saturnian influence here. The unfortunate truth for Lunar Capricorns is that they can struggle with depression or general feelings of melancholy or discontent. Because the Saturnine sense of responsibility weighs heavily upon their shoulders, they may have to work extra hard to break free from their proverbial chains to find the lighter side of life. These people could benefit from learning when to say no, how to stop being so hard on themselves, and when to take a break and experience a bit of fun without feeling guilt. No matter how turbulent their emotions may be under the surface, though, these lunar babes like to keep a tight leash on their feelings and thrive on keeping themselves in check, so you might not be privy to when they're struggling. Capricorns are quite private with their emotions and will only share them with you behind closed doors.

Beyond this, these lovers have a need for strong boundaries and realistic goals. Unlike Lunar Sagittarians, Capricorn Moons are risk-averse, needing a well-thought-out plan and the bounds of safety and security in all areas of their lives in order to function. You can bank on the fact that these lovers have planned well in advance and have thought of damn near everything.

As far as getting their emotional needs met, a Capricorn Moon lover needs to feel worthwhile in the world and their relationships, and they need to feel it in a tangible way. Because they take on so much responsibility, they need not only to be acknowledged and appreciated for their efforts but also to see the results of their hard work playing out in their connections. Respect from others is key for Capricorn more than any other sign. Knowing they have that respect from their loved ones is what feeds their feelings of security and fulfillment, so don't be afraid to tell these lovers just how much respect you have for them!

MOON IN AQUARIUS

Aquarius is one of the more interesting positions of the Moon, in my opinion. The very nature of the fixed air sign of the zodiac is that it is emotionally detached and aloof, much preferring objectivity and practicality in its approach to all things. Whereas the Moon asks for feeling, Aquarius would rather respond with logic. Because of this, Lunar Aquarians, in my experience, tend to greatly struggle with their feelings. Sometimes this struggle can be so great that they often feel they don't understand those feelings— and certainly that nobody else does, either. Of all the air signs in astrology, Aquarius is probably the most guilty of intellectualizing their feelings rather than actually embodying them.

What do I mean by this? Intellectualizing the emotions often involves a great deal of analysis. It's someone who spends a lot of time thinking over what they're going through and picking apart the way they're reacting. This can come across as someone who looks quite self-aware—and in a way they are—but who stops short of actually allowing those feelings to come to the surface and simply exist without having to pick them apart or categorize them. This is especially true with uncomfortable feelings.

Lunar Aquarians prefer to view themselves as being above the baser emotions in life—whatever that means to them—such as jealousy, pettiness, or holding a grudge. Their default is to try and shed whatever emotion they feel isn't serving them and rise above it somehow.

Now, this doesn't mean that Aquarius Moons *don't* struggle with things like jealousy or resentment, but they tend to feel allergic to these very natural emotions! There are lots and lots of lessons for Aquarius around learning to accept and, more importantly, *feel* those feelings, rather than trying to intellectualize them or ignore them altogether.

Beyond this, Aquarius is a rather quirky position of the Moon. The unconventional nature of this sign manifests as unpredictability or a desire to shock in some way, though this may not be readily apparent at first. There is also a surprising amount of pride and stubbornness in these lunar babes. They can become quite cool and fixed in their ways and rebel, rebel, rebel against anyone trying to change or control them.

As a final note, Aquarius Moon lovers make fantastic friends. You can rely on them to show up for the big, important moments in life and to cheer you on unwaveringly, though they may not always be present for the small things, as they need plenty of space, as any good Aquarius does.

Meeting the emotional needs of an Aquarius Moon is all about space, independence, and freedom. These lovers have a wide array of interests, and they need an almost unending amount of time to be able to explore them. The most fulfilling relationships for them will come with people who understand this need, don't take it personally, and will be there whenever Aquarius is ready to come back and share.

MOON IN PISCES

In the final sign of the zodiac, the Moon is especially sensitive—arguably even more sensitive than when the Moon is at home in Cancer. As with all the water sign Moons, the Pisces Moon is incredibly deep and psychic, taking on an impossible amount of emotion and boundlessness. Thanks to the unending amount of empathy that courses through Pisces, someone with this position of the Moon is understanding almost to a fault. There's nothing you can tell a Pisces Moon that they don't understand or resonate with in some way, if for no other reason than their acute psychic senses are enabling them to sense what you're feeling and why.

The ethereal nature of Pisces is amplified through the lens of the Moon, which manifests as a deep struggle to exist in reality. The propensity for delusion, illusion, and fantasy is difficult to overstate and unfortunately makes it difficult for these lovers to see things clearly a lot of the time. In the day-to-day, this makes them a bit flaky. They may struggle to maintain a routine and keep up with the never-ending slog of daily life. Practical affairs and logical savvy are not their strength, but they make up for it in pure intuition and compassion.

Pisces Moon lovers have a soft heart and a sweet nature, granting them the ability to see and understand all the nuances and complexities of what it means to be human. These babes are vivid dreamers, literally and figuratively, and possess an incredible imagination. Because of this, they are likely artistic or creative in some way, even if the rest of the chart doesn't indicate that. This dreamy nature can give them a bit of an absent-minded professor vibe, but it's simply because they are swept up in their daydreams and psychic visions.

Boundaries are hyper important for these lovers, too, as their never-ending acceptance and compassion can make them a bit of a doormat. Learning how to stand up for themselves and establish boundaries without guilt may be a lifelong journey for a Pisces Moon, but it is a necessary one so they don't get bulldozed by less sensitive types. Solitude is something that can be really helpful; a little bit of space to process what they're truly feeling outside of the influence of others' feelings can aid in finding clarity.

As far as feeling nurtured by others, Pisces Moons will fare best in relationships with those who seek to connect on a deep emotional and spiritual level. They, too, require much empathy and understanding and quite frankly need people in their lives who are going to ask them how *they're* doing, too. Pisces placements are notorious for always focusing on other people, often playing the role of therapist, so having supportive relationships with people who recognize their own need to vent is super important. These lovers already know how to give, so they could really benefit from someone who gives back and doesn't require a ton of self-sacrifice on their part.

THE MOON THROUGH THE HOUSES

The house that the Moon, the second luminary, lives in shows the area of our lives where our emotions, and therefore our emotional energy, are wrapped up. We may expend a lot of our emotional energy dealing with the themes of that house, and/or they may have a decided effect on our emotional state. For example, someone with their Moon in the sixth house may be easily affected by their job and whether they had a good day at work or a stressful one, and so on. Their emotions will have a strong impact on their physical health and vice versa.

The associated house of the Moon also points to where we feel the safest and what we need to experience that safety and nurturing. Someone with their Moon in the twelfth house needs lots of alone time and solitude, for example, whereas someone with the Moon in the tenth house needs a stable career to feel secure.

Because the Moon also points to our mom and our relationship with her, we can glean a decent amount of information this way as well. The Moon in the first house can indicate that the person's identity was or is heavily influenced by their mom, whereas the Moon in the twelfth house might indicate the mother being incarcerated or in the hospital or that she's quite intuitive. Really familiarizing yourself with the house your Moon lives in can offer an incredible amount of insight.

Finally, the Moon finds its joy in the third house. In Hellenistic astrology, this house is titled "Goddess," which makes sense, as the Moon has deep roots in being the literal manifestation of the Goddess. The third house is one indication of communication in astrology, and the Moon enjoys being here because it indicates a person who wants to talk about their feelings, which is ultimately what the Moon wants. There can be a tendency to intellectualize the emotions in this house, but that isn't really a bad thing, as it can lead to self-awareness around not only what we're feeling but also what we want and need from others. As these lovers mature, they find a way to balance both their logical and their emotional side.

The Moon in the third house also lends itself to changeability. There is a gift in being able to consider other people's feelings and perspectives as well as one's own and a desire to connect with others on an emotional level. These lovers are likely to base their decision-making on their feelings, and they also need a change of scenery every now and then.

3

MERCURY ☿

DOMICILE: Gemini and Virgo
EXALTATION: Virgo
DETRIMENT: Sagittarius and Pisces
FALL: Pisces

Moving on from the luminaries to Mercury, the first of the actual planets, we again find ourselves in a section of the book that isn't so obviously about sex—at least on the surface. As the planet of communication, Mercury plays an obvious role in romance and, really, relationships of every kind. Communication is one of the most important elements of any relationship and is also an area where people tend to struggle the most. When it comes to exploring and, equally as important, sharing what you want, need, and desire (including in the realm of sex), understanding your Mercurial style can be wildly helpful.

As a quick note, Mercury is the first planet in astrology that experiences retrogrades. Indeed, it is the planet that goes retrograde the most often, thanks to its orbit so close to the Sun, which is contained entirely within the bounds of Earth's orbit. Mercury retrograde has gained quite a reputation for all the ruckus it stirs up during these transits. The trouble is so noticeable that Mercury retrograde has transcended the boundaries of the astrologically inclined and just about everyone talks about it!

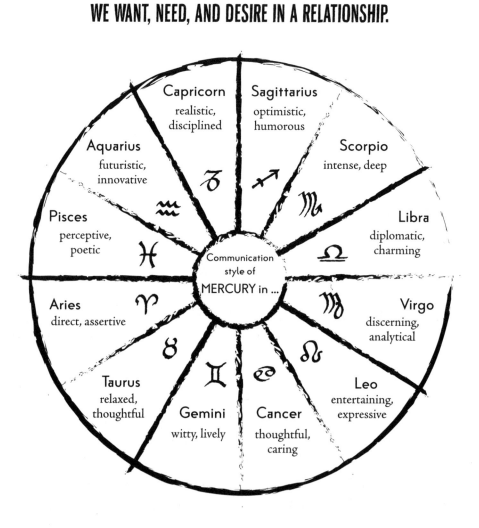

MERCURY POINTS TO HOW WE COMMUNICATE WHAT WE WANT, NEED, AND DESIRE IN A RELATIONSHIP.

Communication style of MERCURY in ...

Capricorn
realistic, disciplined

Sagittarius
optimistic, humorous

Scorpio
intense, deep

Aquarius
futuristic, innovative

Libra
diplomatic, charming

Pisces
perceptive, poetic

Virgo
discerning, analytical

Aries
direct, assertive

Leo
entertaining, expressive

Taurus
relaxed, thoughtful

Gemini
witty, lively

Cancer
thoughtful, caring

I bring this up because, as we move forward, it is highly possible that you may be someone who has retrograde planets in your birth chart. This is a question that often gets brought up in my consultations with clients. Whenever we see a planet that is retrograde in the natal chart, the nature of that planet tends to express itself more internally than normal, which is to say this energy may show up as a person being more introverted or introspective than we would normally expect. Take it from me: I have my natal Mercury in Virgo, which is both at home and exalted and is normally a super chatty placement! However, it's also retrograde in my chart, and I am definitely an introvert. I often need to step away to really reflect on things and formulate my words carefully.

There is also something a bit unexpected about natally retrograde planets. Where Mercury is concerned, for example, those who were born during a retrograde tend to fare quite well during the retrograde transits and may even find greater ease during those times. I think it's something important to consider as we move forward through this book.

MERCURY IN ARIES

Anybody with their Mercury in the first sign of the zodiac embodies and desires direct communication. Mercury in Aries gives individuals a dynamic, assertive approach to communication and thinking. Bordering on being downright blunt, an Aries Mercury isn't afraid to speak their mind. They're going to tell you exactly what they want, both in and out of the bedroom. As a rule, Aries placements are bold. You will always know exactly where you stand with these lovers, as they are going to voice exactly what they think and how they feel. They speak their mind without hesitation and are not afraid to state their opinions or take charge of a conversation. Aries is not afraid to stand up for themselves, to get into an argument if necessary, or to tell someone where to stick it.

Those with Mercury in Aries have a sharp and quick-witted intellect, with the ability to think on their feet and respond rapidly to new information or challenges. Because of this, they thrive in fast-paced environments where they can take decisive action.

The way an Aries Mercury speaks is passionate, too. Their speech can become loud when they are excited, and there is something infectious and hilarious about them. The beauty of this position of Mercury is that they will stand up for you, too, if you need them to—and sometimes even if you don't!

Mercury in Aries individuals may have a tendency to act impulsively or make snap decisions without fully considering the consequences, preferring to trust their instincts. They may not always take the time to weigh all the options. They thrive on taking risks and pushing boundaries in pursuit of their goals. Even with Mercury, Aries possesses a competitive streak, channeling this energy into intellectual debates or competitions. They thrive on the adrenaline rush of competition and may be drawn to careers that allow them to showcase their intellect and leadership skills, though Aries does value their independence and may prefer to work alone rather than on a team. They are self-reliant individuals who trust their own judgment and instincts above all else.

Mercury in Aries individuals tend to have a short attention span, getting bored easily, and may quickly lose interest in topics that do not stimulate their intellect or excite their passion. Aries thrives on novelty and excitement and will constantly seek out new challenges to keep themselves engaged. At the end of the day, Mercury in Aries individuals possess a dynamic and assertive intellect, with a focus on taking action and pursuing their goals with courage and determination. As the first cardinal sign, they are natural leaders and innovators who are not afraid to blaze their own trail in pursuit of success.

MERCURY IN TAURUS

In a stark departure from the fiery nature of Aries, a Taurus Mercury is incredibly chill. Mercury in this sign gives these individuals a grounded and deliberate approach to communication and thinking. Their mental energy is tied up in the practical, and they can be extremely focused on their goals, especially the ones involving money. As is typical of Taurus, these people may have a strong focus on material possessions and financial security. They value stability and may be drawn to careers that offer a steady income and opportunities for advancement.

As far as conversation is concerned, these people tend to be relaxed. A Mercury in Taurus communicates in a steady and deliberate manner. They choose their words carefully and prefer to speak slowly and thoughtfully rather than rushing their speech. Thanks to being the first earth sign, they also have a practical and down-to-earth mindset, focusing on tangible results and concrete solutions to problems. In Taurus, Mercury has a patient and methodical approach to problem-solving, taking the time to carefully consider all the options before making a decision. They are skilled at applying logic and reason rather than emotions to their decision-making process.

One thing to keep in mind is that a Taurus Mercury has incredibly strong convictions. Because Taurus is the sign associated with values, people with this Mercury placement know exactly what theirs are. When combined with the bull's resistance to change, they are unlikely to waver once they have formed an opinion or made a decision, even in the face of new information. And thanks to this sign's impeccable stubborn streak, it may be damn near impossible to change their mind!

Mercury in Taurus has a sensual and tactile communication style, often using descriptive language that appeals to the senses. These individuals appreciate beauty and may have a talent for expressing themselves through art, music, or other creative mediums.

More than anything else, Mercury in Taurus folks are resilient and dependable and can be relied on to follow through on their commitments. They have a strong work ethic and are willing to put in the effort required to achieve their goals. Remember that Taurus's stubborn nature, when channeled correctly, blooms into a steadfastness unrivaled and unmatched by any other sign.

MERCURY IN GEMINI

The planet of communication finds its first home here with the cosmic twins. Geminis are known for being incredibly talkative, and this is especially true—perhaps the most true even—when Mercury is here, in domicile. Thanks to its home field position, Mercury's intellectual prowess is heightened in Aries, creating people who know a lot about a lot and are sharp, witty, and lively. Geminis are fucking smart and wield a sharp, agile intellect. They are quick thinkers who excel at processing information rapidly and making connections between different ideas. This versatility also gets channeled into their communication style: Gemini is skilled at expressing themselves in a variety of ways, including writing, speaking, and using nonverbal cues. They have a charming communication style that draws others to them. They are witty and entertaining conversationalists who know how to keep people engaged with their words.

Mercury in Gemini has a natural curiosity and thirst for knowledge. These individuals enjoy learning about a wide range of topics and may have a tendency to jump from one subject to another in pursuit of new information.

Mercury in Gemini's tendency to jump from one topic to the next to the next can be their downfall, however, as they often wind up feeling interested in everything and therefore nothing and can struggle greatly to commit to any one thing. This is true for all Gemini placements and can cause them great unease throughout their lives. Learning to embrace this part of themselves and see it as a gift rather than a curse can set them free.

One of the best parts about having a Gemini Mercury is that it gives these lovers the ability to understand virtually every perspective. This is a handy quality to have when it comes to relationships, as Gemini can and will put themselves in another person's shoes, able to understand why and how a person is feeling. In fact, Gemini is the most adept at understanding where other people are coming from, especially if it's something more logic-based, though that doesn't mean feelings are outside their wheelhouse. This superpower enables Gemini to connect with others easily, which is ultimately what they're looking to do.

MERCURY IN CANCER

Those with Mercury in nurturing, doting Cancer tend to be quite sweet. In this sign, Mercury combines the intellectual with the emotional, creating a person with an empathetic, intuitive, and caring communication style. Certainly those with a Cancer Mercury command a strong emotional intelligence, able to easily read and attune themselves to the feelings of others. These are the therapist friends of the zodiac, who spend a lot of time listening to the emotions of those around them. Their comforting, understanding communication style makes them feel like a safe haven to their loved ones. Their fiercely protective nature further cultivates feelings of safety and security in their relationships, fostering the trust others need to open up.

The flip side of this is that people with Mercury in Cancer are also adept at sharing their own feelings and possess an incredible memory, especially when it comes to experiences that have a strong emotional connection. They are deep thinkers and take their time in responding to others or situations, acting from a careful, intentional place. Cancer is a deeply reflective and spiritual sign, and through the lens of Mercury, it makes these individuals quite thoughtful and rather quiet. They much prefer one-on-one interactions over groups or crowds.

The sensitive, moody nature of Mercury in Cancer can make these lovers a bit defensive in conversation, however, as the instinct to protect themselves is strong. They can also get their feelings hurt quite easily. Whenever this happens, these lovers are going to withdraw, sucking themselves up into the safety of their crabby shell to lick their wounds. And trust me, there's no pulling them back *out* of that shell until they are good and ready! Ultimately, these lovers aren't looking for a fight—though that doesn't mean they won't fight you if they have to—and are more likely to shut down and isolate.

With Mercury in Cancer, everything gets filtered through the lens of the emotions, even if other placements in the chart point to a more logical or practical disposition. Cancer gets frustrated by a facts-only approach, as this tends to undermine the very real influence of the emotions and doesn't take into account any of the nuances or complexities of a situation. These lovers are adept at unraveling those pieces of a situation and can intuit an incredible amount of information.

MERCURY IN LEO

When Mercury is in Leo, it takes on qualities that are bold, expressive, and confident. Individuals with Mercury in this sign tend to communicate in a dramatic and expressive manner, and they often have a flair for storytelling and can captivate an audience with their words—and their hands! As with other Leo placements, there's a natural confidence in how people with Mercury in Leo communicate. They are not afraid to speak their mind and can be quite assertive in expressing their opinions and ideas. Mercury in Leo also fosters creativity and original thinking. These individuals often have a unique perspective and enjoy exploring innovative ideas.

Naturally, those with Mercury in Leo enjoy being the center of attention and can command a room with their presence, as Leo is a natural leader. They speak from the heart and are passionate about what they believe in. This enthusiasm can be quite contagious and even inspiring to those around them. And while Leo can be self-centered, a Leo Mercury tends to be generous with praise and compliments, recognizing the efforts and achievements of others openly and enthusiastically.

That said, Mercury in Leo individuals *do* thrive on attention and recognition. They enjoy being admired for their intellect, unique perspectives, charisma, and communication skills (or anything else you might like about them). Ultimately, a Leo Mercury is not afraid to take charge and often excels in roles where they can influence and motivate others.

When it comes to sex, Mercury in Leo wants to hear just how sexy you think they are. Remember, they thrive on compliments, so they're looking to hear just how good all their sexual skills are—maybe even compared to other lovers. Don't worry, though—Leo is just as generous when it comes to giving compliments, so they'll be sure to tell you all the things you do well in return.

MERCURY IN VIRGO

Virgo is a special placement for Mercury, as it is the only sign where we see Mercury both at home and in its exaltation. Mercury is unique in this way, too, as we don't come across any other planet in astrology that is both at home and exalted in the same sign. And while it's true that Virgo can be quite talkative, the energy a Virgo Mercury embodies is much different from when Mercury is at home in its other sign, Gemini. This is likely due, at least in part, to Virgo being an earth sign and not an air sign. By nature, there is a much more grounded coloring to Virgo, making those with this Mercury placement more reserved and intentional with their words. Mercury in Virgo folks possess a keen intellect and an analytical mind. They thrive on critical thinking and are highly organized, detail-oriented, and exacting.

Now, that critical nature is a hallmark for Mercury here. Unfortunately, Virgo has garnered a reputation for being too critical of others and sharp with their words. It's true that Virgo isn't one to sugarcoat things and their delivery isn't always wrapped up in a pretty bow. However, despite how they may come off, these individuals are truly coming from a place of wanting to help. I promise you these lovers have spent some time analyzing the situation, and because they are gifted with the ability to see the most efficient path forward, they are coming to you armed with the best solution.

When it comes to the topic of sex, those with Mercury in Virgo can be a bit shy or uncomfortable voicing the things they like or want done to them. You won't find them dishing about their sexual escapades, either. It's simply not in their nature. However, once a Virgo Mercury gets comfortable with someone, you might be surprised just how dirty that mouth can be.

MERCURY IN LIBRA

With Mercury in the sign of scales, we see someone who truly values open and balanced communication. Mercury in Libra imbues individuals with a communicative style that emphasizes harmony and diplomacy. The main way this manifests is through wanting an even give-and-take in their conversations with others. For example, if a Libra asks, "How are you?," a response such as "good" without the follow-up of "You?" is the kiss of death. This need for balance in conversations is further fueled by Libra's penchant for tactfulness and manners. To them, it's just plain rude not to ask someone how they're doing in return.

Individuals with Mercury in Libra have a natural talent for diplomacy. They strive to maintain balance in their interactions and are skilled at finding common ground in discussions. Because Libras are so adept at seeing both sides of an issue, this position of Mercury makes a person a fantastic mediator or negotiator, possessing the ability to help foster compromise and to find solutions that work for everyone. These people value fairness and justice in communication and are often advocates for equality and equity.

As with all Libra placements, individuals with Mercury here possess a certain charm. They have a way with words that can win over others and smooth over conflicts with grace and finesse. They excel in social situations and are skilled at building rapport with a wide range of people. They also enjoy engaging in intellectual conversations and are often sought after for their insights and advice. As Mercury in Libra has a keen aesthetic sensibility and appreciates beauty in language and communication, these folks may have a talent for poetry, writing, or other forms of artistic expression.

These lovers value collaboration and are willing to compromise to maintain harmony in relationships. And, yes, despite their ability to see both sides of an issue, Mercury in Libra individuals can sometimes struggle with indecision, as they weigh the pros and cons of various options before making a decision.

In the bedroom, Mercury in Libra is looking for an even give-and-take. While their default is to please, and therefore they'll want to know what their lovers want or like, at a certain point they're going to need to be asked what they want, too. Without this consideration shown in return, a Libra Mercury will lose interest or shut down.

MERCURY IN SCORPIO

In deep, dark, and intense Scorpio, Mercury gifts these individuals with a sharp, probing intellect and incredible mental fortitude. People with Mercury in Scorpio have a keen intuition and are skilled at uncovering hidden truths and underlying motivations. They have a way of seeing through all the fluff and cutting straight to the heart of a situation or individual. Their ability to really see someone can be unnerving for some.

People with Mercury in Scorpio possess a sharp intellect that allows them to delve beneath the surface and understand complex issues on a deeper level. They have a strong will and are not afraid to confront difficult or taboo subjects. They can handle intense mental challenges and are often drawn to topics related to psychology, mysticism, or the occult. The communication style of a Scorpio Mercury is direct, assertive, and sometimes intense. These individuals are not afraid to speak their mind and can be quite persuasive when they are passionate about a topic.

Those with Mercury in Scorpio also excel at research and investigation. They have a natural curiosity and enjoy uncovering secrets and solving mysteries or puzzles. They are adept at gathering information and analyzing data to uncover hidden patterns or truths. More than any other position of Mercury, these individuals wield a detective-like mindset and are skilled at ferreting out lies and deception. They can see through superficiality and are not easily fooled by others' manipulative tactics. Scorpios are the FBI detectives who are going to solve the crime.

Beyond this, those with a Scorpio Mercury have a rich emotional life and are deeply attuned to the feelings of themselves and others. They may have a tendency to brood or dwell on intense emotions, but they also have the ability to transform emotional pain into personal growth. Despite this, Mercury in Scorpio individuals value their privacy and may be secretive about their own thoughts and feelings. They prefer to keep their cards close to their chest and may not reveal everything they know or suspect.

When thinking about the way a Scorpio Mercury shows up in the bedroom, it can be a bit complex. Because of their private ways, they don't typically kiss and tell. It's more likely that a Scorpio Mercury will *show* you how much they want you rather than tell you. Remember that it takes them a while to trust and open up, but once they do, they have a wicked mouth.

MERCURY IN SAGITTARIUS

In Jupiter-ruled Sagittarius, Mercury is in the first sign of its detriment. This is perhaps a bit ironic, as Sagittarius dons the title of the truth seeker in astrology. Nevertheless, we find Mercury feeling quite uncomfortable here.

The reason for this is that Mercury thrives in the details and Sagittarius is about the big picture—which is to say the exact opposite of Mercury. Where Mercury seeks to learn, Sagittarius seeks to teach and preach. The two-way nature of communication gives way to the one-sided energy of Sag, who wishes to impart the knowledge they possess to others. While there is a time and place for such things, these individuals tend to bring that energy to any and all of their conversations, which can make them overbearing, inflammatory, and unwilling to learn or compromise. Despite the mutable nature of Sagittarius, those with this Mercury placement tend to think their beliefs are the right way and the only way, and therefore they can struggle to listen and consider other perspectives.

The flip side of this is that Mercury in Sagittarius lovers are full of *big* ideas. They are optimistic and hilarious and have a vision. They can be restless in the intellectual sense, as they are forward-thinking, and get easily frustrated or bogged down in details. They want to focus on the bigger topics in life, such as religion, spirituality, and philosophy, and are decidedly turned off by dry subjects and small talk. They need lots of room for freethinking and turning over the bigger questions about life. They'd rather have a hot debate or discuss heady topics with their partners than discuss what needs to be purchased at the grocery store.

With Mercury in this fire sign, these lovers are pretty bold. It's unlikely that a Sagittarius Mercury will have any trouble letting you know that they want you. Humor is a huge turn-on for them, so being able to joke and make them laugh will serve you well. It's likely that they, too, will tease you as a way of flirting. These lovers are also attracted to accents and foreign languages.

MERCURY IN CAPRICORN

In Capricorn, Mercury instills a person with a practical, disciplined, and strategic approach to communication and thinking. Individuals with Mercury in Capricorn have a practical and realistic mindset. They approach problems from a rational and logical perspective, focusing on finding tangible solutions rather than getting caught up in abstract concepts, as we see with all earth signs. They are systematic and organized in their communication and have a knack for breaking down complex ideas into manageable steps and presenting them in a clear and concise manner.

As with all Capricorn placements, Mercury in this sign is ambitious and goal-oriented. We see people who expend much of their mental energy focusing on said goals and how to achieve them. Those with a Capricorn Mercury have a strong sense of purpose and are willing to work hard to achieve their objectives. They are strategic in their planning and are not easily deterred by obstacles or setbacks. They follow through on their commitments and expect others to do the same.

Typically, those with Mercury in Capricorn have respect for tradition and may have a more conservative approach to communication and thinking. We can see this most readily through the Capricorn value of stability; they may be resistant to change unless they see a clear benefit. They have a natural aptitude for business and may excel in careers that require strategic thinking and decision-making.

Unsurprisingly, Mercury in Capricorn individuals can be reserved or cautious in their expression, preferring to think things through carefully before speaking. They may not be the most spontaneous or expressive communicators, but they are reliable and trustworthy. They have a patient and disciplined approach to everything and are willing to invest the time and effort required to reach their objectives in all areas.

MERCURY IN AQUARIUS

Personally, I think Mercury is fantastic in Aquarius. Uranus, the modern-day ruler of Aquarius, also rules over the higher mind and represents our unique inner genius. Therefore, in my opinion, Mercury does quite well here—even if these individuals tend to think about things or harbor certain ideas and perspectives that the rest of us might not quite understand. Regardless, Mercury in Aquarius gives a person a unique, innovative, and intellectually curious mindset.

Those with Mercury in Aquarius have a highly original and unconventional approach to thinking. They are creative and innovative and often come up with unique solutions to problems that others may not have considered.

In Aquarius, the sign of the dissemination of knowledge, Mercury is constantly seeking new information and ideas. People with Mercury here enjoy exploring a wide range of topics and may have eclectic interests that span multiple fields of study. They are forward-thinking, progressive, highly open-minded individuals who are receptive to new ideas, and they enjoy engaging in intellectually stimulating conversations with others.

Through the Mercurial lens, we most obviously see the objective and detached perspective that Aquarius is famous for. This allows individuals with Mercury in Aquarius to analyze situations with clarity and impartiality. They are not swayed by emotions or personal biases when making decisions, preferring instead to approach things from a purely logical place.

Those with an Aquarius Mercury have a unique and quirky communication style that sets them apart from others. They may use humor, sarcasm, or irony to make their point, and they enjoy challenging conventional wisdom and questioning authority. As with all Aquarius placements, Mercury in this sign has a rebellious streak and may be drawn to countercultural movements or alternative lifestyles. These folks are not afraid to challenge the status quo and may enjoy pushing boundaries and breaking free from societal norms.

Mercury in Aquarius individuals are often driven by a sense of social justice and a desire to make the world a better place. They are passionate about causes that promote equality, freedom, and individual rights. They have a futuristic outlook and are interested in exploring the possibilities of what the future may hold. Those with an Aquarius Mercury may be drawn to fields such as technology, science fiction, or futurism. Overall, these individuals possess a highly intellectual and visionary mindset, with a focus on innovation, progress, and social change. They are natural thinkers and communicators who are always looking ahead to what lies beyond the horizon.

MERCURY IN PISCES

The planet of communication is said to be in detriment in watery Pisces, the opposite sign of Virgo, one of Mercury's domains. Mercury in Pisces is sometimes described as being mute in Pisces, and people with this natal placement may struggle to communicate exactly what they're thinking or feeling, as it can be hard for them to pin down or it may feel like it changes from one minute to the next. Mercury in Pisces has a sensitive, imaginative, and intuitive approach to communication and thinking. These individuals have a vivid imagination and a rich inner world. They are creative and intuitive thinkers who often come up with innovative ideas and solutions. Thanks to their powerful imagination, their communication style can be dreamy and poetic, with a tendency to speak in metaphors or symbols. They have a gift for storytelling and may excel in creative writing or other forms of artistic expression.

Mercury in Pisces lovers are empathetic, compassionate, and full of understanding, preferring to focus on other people and their emotions, ready to help them process what they're going through. Understanding the emotions and perspectives of others is a Pisces superpower, making these individuals excellent listeners and counselors.

Those with a Pisces Mercury have a strong intuitive sense and may rely on gut feelings or instincts when making decisions. They are attuned to subtle energies and may pick up on things that others overlook, detecting subtle cues or vibes from others. Because they are hypersensitive, they may need to retreat into solitude occasionally to recharge their emotional batteries.

Individuals with Mercury in Pisces tend to have a nonlinear thinking process and may have difficulty with logical reasoning at times. This isn't to say they are incapable of seeing logic, but their baseline is rooted in their emotions and they will always default to making choices based on their feelings first. They may prefer to see the big picture rather than getting bogged down in details.

In true Piscean fashion, folks with Mercury in this sign have a deep spiritual awareness and may be drawn to mystical or metaphysical subjects. They are interested in exploring the mysteries of the universe and may have a strong connection to their inner spiritual guidance. Again, as is true with all Pisces placements, Mercury in Pisces may have a tendency to escape from reality through daydreaming, fantasy, or creative pursuits. These individuals may struggle with practical matters or have difficulty staying grounded in the here and now. Truly, though, they are natural dreamers and visionaries who are able to tap into the deeper currents of the human experience.

When it comes to sex, Mercury in Pisces lovers want soft talk. Anything brash or uncouth will have them withering on the vine. However, keep in mind that these folks love a good fantasy, so role-playing is a good, fun way to get them to open up.

A NOTE ON THE HOUSES

The next layer of understanding Mercury in the chart comes from exploring the house it resides in. The themes of the appropriate house point to the sort of topics the person spends a lot of time thinking about or discussing—similar to the way that the sign Mercury is in does—and potentially whom they like to converse with. For example, someone with their Mercury in the fourth house may spend a lot of time thinking about their families, their ancestors, the things they were taught as a child, and so on, and they may just enjoy talking with their family members, period. Someone with their Mercury in the eleventh house may have an interest in technology, social media, and looking toward the future. You get the idea. The house containing Mercury can also be a place of travel or busyness, as Mercury rules over our movements in the day-to-day, as well as where we like to show up and express ourselves the most.

Continuing on with our discussion of planetary joys, for Mercury that title belongs to the first house. The first house is called "the Helm," as in the helm of a ship. One of the traditional associations of Mercury is travel and commerce, so we see an intuitive connection here.

As with everything contained in the first house, a person with this house position of Mercury readily embodies its busy, communicative energy. These lovers will certainly be chatty, loving to engage in conversation with any and everyone around them. They are open and honest in their communication and love to share their thoughts with others.

Especially in the first house of identity, Mercury here will have a strong desire (or perhaps a downright need) to share who they are. Candid self-expression is key here, as is having relationships with those who value their perspectives. Those with Mercury in the first house will want to share their thoughts and feelings on all things, sometimes to no end, so they will fare best with people who share the same values around communication. These lovers want to be seen *and* heard, though there may be some lessons for them to learn around active listening!

Because being able to share both their identity and their beliefs is important to them, lovers with Mercury in the first house have no trouble standing up for and asserting themselves. They have no qualms about speaking their mind and telling their partners exactly what they're looking for, both in and out of the bedroom (depending on other placements in the birth chart, of course).

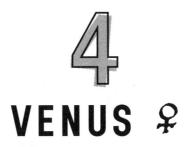

VENUS ♀

DOMICILE: Taurus and Libra

EXALTATION: Pisces

DETRIMENT: Scorpio and Aries

FALL: Virgo

Immortalized in the heavens as the goddess of love and beauty, Venus is the main partnership planet in astrology. Although Mars, her counterpart, also grapples with themes of relationships (which we will cover in the next chapter), Venus represents the quintessential ideals of love and romance. Often thought of as the feminine principle of partnership—which is to say the passive, receptive side—Venus represents the archetype of the lover that we embody. It characterizes the way we love and the things we value and are attracted to in partners and partnerships and can also inform our aesthetic sensibilities. Every beautiful thing that moves us, every piece of art we admire or create or marvel at, is symbolized by Venus. Our musical tastes, our sense of style, the types of landscapes we think are prettiest, and the people we find attractive are all informed by Venus. There is a popular line of thought in astrology that we can dial up our personal magnetism by dressing for our Venus sign. The way we choose to dress and style our hair and the accessories we choose to adorn ourselves with—or not—are directly linked to Venus. Through physically embodying the style of our Venus placement, we are more easily able to attract the things and people we desire.

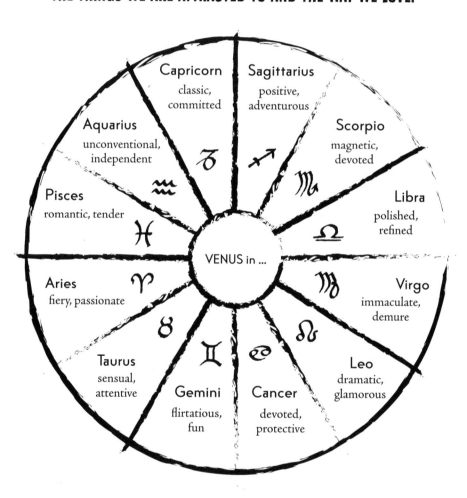

VENUS IS THE MAIN PARTNERSHIP PLANET
AND REPRESENTS LOVE AND ROMANCE. IT CHARACTERIZES
THE THINGS WE ARE ATTRACTED TO AND THE WAY WE LOVE.

VENUS in ...

Capricorn
classic, committed

Sagittarius
positive, adventurous

Aquarius
unconventional, independent

Scorpio
magnetic, devoted

Pisces
romantic, tender

Libra
polished, refined

Aries
fiery, passionate

Virgo
immaculate, demure

Taurus
sensual, attentive

Leo
dramatic, glamorous

Gemini
flirtatious, fun

Cancer
devoted, protective

Regardless of our gender, Venus graces us all with her gifts one way or another. We are all lovers under her seductive charms, defenseless against her intoxicating promise. Everything, everything, everything is Venus.

As the eternal rose that embodies love itself, Venus is one of the principal placements we look to in sextrology to start unraveling and understanding the essence of our sexual and romantic nature. As sex and romance often go hand in hand, it's crucial not only to know what you desire in your relationships but also to have an awareness around how you show up. Remember that relationships are symbiotic, and it takes more than one person to make things work. In that sense, as a sidenote on compatibility, it is invaluable to understand your loved one's Venus placement as well. And while, yes, there definitely are certain placements that have an easier time together, remember that Venus (or any planet, for that matter) is only one piece of the pie. However, especially where romantic connections are concerned, Venus comes forward to play a much more dominant role than usual.

VENUS IN ARIES

Here in Aries, the first sign of the zodiac, Venus is said to be in its detriment, as Aries is the sign opposite Libra, one of Venus's home signs. Whenever a planet is in detriment, it's believed to struggle in that sign and thus—in this case—in love and partnerships. Don't let this discourage you, however! My Venus is in detriment (in Scorpio, in my case), and it's my favorite placement in my entire chart.

Aries is cardinal fire energy and is therefore the sign of the self. It's also a Mars-ruled sign and gives the feminine energy of Venus a much more masculine edge. However, Aries is also the archetype of the warrior and the leader and is therefore a fierce defender of all matters of the heart.

Thanks to the fiery nature of Aries, Venus in this sign is incredibly passionate. It's one of the most passionate placements for Venus, in fact, and for these individuals there's a strong need for their partners to be able to match their level of ardor. Aries is a physical sign, period, and needs—perhaps more than most—to express this passion physically.

That's right—people with an Aries Venus are horny as hell. They like to do it and do it often. Thanks to the natural vitality that Aries placements bring, this makes for an incredible vigor that's always ready to go. It may be difficult for these lovers to find a partner who can keep up! However, it's deeply important for anybody with this placement to unabashedly own this part of themselves. In fact, it is the key to sexual empowerment for these creatures—as well as to own the fact that anybody who can't match them on both an emotional and a physical level when it comes to the flames of desire just isn't going to work.

Once the match has been lit, Venus in Aries is all in and extremely loyal. These people are extremely clear about what and who they want, and they won't waste any time beating around the bush. For an Aries Venus, there is always a sense of urgency, making these lovers direct, bold, and up-front about their feelings and intentions. They can also be protective, territorial, and jealous, as well as dominant both in and out of the bedroom. However, without the proportional fuel from a potential counterpart, that flame can die out just as quickly, and Aries is out the door.

In order to establish and maintain emotional intimacy, Venus in Aries needs a partner who is unyieldingly demonstrative in their feelings. An Aries Venus will always appreciate clear and consistent words and actions from their partner, letting them know exactly where their heart lies. The energy of Aries wants to be out and moving in the world, so a partner with an equal measure of fun who is down to ride is also important.

As Aries is the sign of the self, though, there are definitely lessons surrounding compromise for those with this Venus placement. Our partner's feelings, wants, needs, and perspectives are just as valuable as our own, and learning how and when to prioritize those is an invaluable lesson for all of us. However, this is especially true for anyone with a fire sign Venus.

Keys to Empowerment

With your Venus in Aries, there is a need, first and foremost, to own exactly what you're looking for in a partner. Aries is always extremely clear about what and who they want and need. Why lie to yourself about what that is?

The rest of us should be so lucky to have such pointed clarity in matters of love and sex.

I think it's also important to recognize that as you grow and change, so will your needs and wishes. Perhaps it's time to revisit this concept. What do you absolutely need from a partner? What do you want? What are you willing to compromise on and where will you absolutely not compromise?

Beyond this, with Venus in Aries, the sign of the self, you absolutely require relationships where you can be completely yourself and find love, respect, and acceptance for this. In sex, specifically, there's a need to own—and be able to do—exactly what you want. This isn't an invitation to be a selfish lover, but rather to know that sexual empowerment starts first within yourself. Passion and desire burn hot in Aries placements. With your Venus in Aries, certainly your partner needs to match this fervor and understand your inherent need to express your feelings through physical connection, but remember that we all spend time alone in this life. How can you embody and engage with your sexuality all by yourself?

VENUS IN TAURUS

Venus is at home in Taurus. It is said to be in domicile in this sign and feels extremely at ease here. Since Taurus is an earth sign, there is something incredibly grounding about the nature of love that a person with this placement possesses. Their partners may view them as an unwavering source of solace and support, someone they can depend on without question time and again.

Getting a Taurus Venus to become your lover in the first place, however, is a very different story. People with Venus in this sign are extremely slow-moving when it comes to love. These lovers are the people who will hang out with someone *every day* for months without ever making a move. Taurus is notoriously slow to do pretty much everything, and Venus here is no exception. A Taurus Venus feels much more comfortable slowly wiggling their way into someone's heart than diving in headfirst. A feeling of safety is of the utmost importance to them and is a crucial element for empowerment in intimacy, both sexually and emotionally.

For those with Venus in Taurus, safety is usually established through a good routine within the relationship. These lovers thrive on stability—and, more importantly, predictability. These are the people who actually enjoy a bit of monotony in their partnerships and are more apt to want to hang out at home than go on some spontaneous adventure. For those who are looking to move faster in love, Venus in Taurus can be maddening, allowing everything about the relationship to move at an almost glacial pace. The flip side of this is that these folks make stable partners who are here for both a good time and a long time.

Due to the earthy energy of Venus in Taurus, people with this placement are incredibly sensual lovers. They like to take a hands-on approach to love, valuing physical touch and affection—as well as quality time. Just as with everything else in life, a Taurus Venus likes to take their time once in the bedroom.

Venus in Taurus lovers are also incredibly focused on the person of their affections and will pay attention to every little detail about them. They are likely to gift you that thing you mentioned you wanted in passing one time but totally forgot about. Thanks to the material indulgence that we see with Taurus, lovers with Venus in this sign will want to experience opulence and luxury in their relationships as well. Think expensive dinners and Gucci sweaters.

Keys to Empowerment

Whenever we look at Venus in domicile, we look at the concept of indulgence. As an earth sign, Taurus thrives on anything that engages the five senses. Things need to look, feel, smell, taste, and sound good to them. Taurus also loves to take its time.

This is an inherently sensual sign. Taurus lives deep in the realm of pleasure. Yes, of course, we're talking about sex, but pleasure encompasses so much more than that. With this Venus placement, it's important to seek out things that stimulate unbridled pleasure.

With your Venus in Taurus, relish every bite. Take a four-hour bubble bath. Enjoy the feel of fresh sheets. You get the idea. There is a freedom to be found through guilt-free indulgence. What sparks those sensations for you? How can you cultivate that experience both solo and in your romantic connections?

Taurus is also associated with safety, stability, and predictability, and Venus in Taurus tends to trend toward monogamy and commitment rather than casual sex (which isn't to say that never happens!). Trust goes hand in hand with safety, and it starts with feeling safe in your own body. Do you feel safe in your body and in your surrounding environment? If not, it's time to look at what you need in order to feel that way. If you can't feel secure in your physical vessel, there's no way you'll be able to extend that feeling when interacting with someone else. Remember that Taurus loves to take things slow, and it's okay if you need to take things slow both with yourself and with someone else.

VENUS IN GEMINI

In busy Gemini, Venus takes on a very different tone than when it's in Aries or Taurus. No longer in either detriment or domicile, Venus strikes out into new territory when it's in Gemini.

In airy Gemini, Venus is fun and full of life. People with this placement love to go out and actually *do* things with their love interests, as they're always looking for (mental) stimulation and ways to stay engaged, preferring to keep things light and flirtatious during their many activities. This isn't to say that Venus in Gemini is incapable of going deep. On the contrary, they value open and honest communication above all else. But this position of the planet of love is notoriously difficult to pin down. Those with Venus in Gemini tend to get bored easily and are just as quick to leave as they are to jump in. Winning and keeping the attention of a Venus in Gemini lover is no easy task. However, on the rare occasion that someone does manage to capture their undivided attention, Gemini is ready to go all in.

As the first of the mutable signs, Gemini loves variety. We can see this through the many different lovers and various love affairs of those with Venus in Gemini. Someone with this position of Venus can go through many different flings, situationships, and committed relationships. Thanks to

Gemini's love of variety, this is the first position of Venus where we can see someone who may be open to, well, open relationships. The gift of mutability means that Gemini is open to trying all different approaches and can see the value of trying on all kinds of relationship styles. In my experience with clients and people in general, whenever Venus is transiting Gemini, like clockwork, people start toying with the idea of opening up their relationships and exploring polyamory!

A Gemini Venus may not appear to have a "type" as much as others do, at least as far as looks are concerned. The key component of attraction for them lies within a person's intelligence. Again, Venus in Gemini has to find a person *interesting*—they can't be just any Joe Schmo off the street. Typically, a Gemini Venus also wants to keep the relationship light. As much as they're willing to discuss all manner of things, a partner (or relationship) that is too overdone will cause them to wither on the vine.

Now, thanks to Mercury being the ruling planet of Gemini, communication doesn't stop at the threshold of the bedroom for these folks. A Gemini Venus can be quite vocal in the bedroom. They may like dirty talk or someone who is just as emotive in bed as they are. Venus here also loves oral sex! Anything involving the mouth is a yes. Their love of variety also translates into someone who is adventurous in the bedroom. They are down for a good time, a long time, a quickie, having sex in the bedroom, the bathroom, outside—you name it. Again we see Gemini's desire for fun and the need for a partner who is down to ride.

Keys to Empowerment

There is a need, first and foremost, for any Venus in Gemini lover to own their need for open and honest communication. Difficult as this may be for many signs, Gemini has no problem here. Someone who is avoidant in this way or doesn't share the same values around communication will ultimately be the kiss of death for a Gemini Venus. In my experience, finding a partner who matches their communicative nature is often a struggle for these lovers, but whenever they let that need fall to the wayside, they inevitably end up feeling deflated and unfulfilled. If you have Venus in Gemini, what would it look like to wait to get involved with someone until you know they are ready, willing, and able to meet you here? What would it mean to find a partner— or partners—who values open, honest, and constant communication the way you do?

Intellectual foreplay is a must for a Gemini Venus, and there's simply no reason to compromise here. You might like to think of people with this Venus placement as sapiosexual: smart people who are hot. For Venus in Gemini, nothing gets the juices flowing like someone who can stimulate your mind before they stimulate anything else.

VENUS IN CANCER

In the sign of the crab, Venus takes up its first watery position in the salty ocean—an interesting connection, in my humble opinion, as in myth, Venus was born from the sea!

Tender and nurturing Venus in Cancer searches for a deep emotional connection in their relationships. Like pretty much every other placement in this cardinal water sign, Venus here thrives on emotional intelligence and being able to connect on an almost purely emotional level. They crave knowing all the nooks and crannies of their loved ones and being able to openly express feelings on both (or all) sides of the table. In fact, this kind of connection is the most important as far as Cancer is concerned. Remember that safety, trust, and emotional intimacy are the bread and butter of any kind of relationship for a Cancer Venus, and without it, the connection won't go very far.

At first these lovers are quite guarded with their emotions. Armed with a crabby shell and razor-sharp claws, a Venus in Cancer's instincts will always be to protect their soft, squishy heart that lies inside. Because of this, it may take them a while to open up. They will likely take their time observing a person, needing to interact with them a few times in order to weigh whether or not that person *feels* safe, whether or not it's worth it to bother opening up to them. Once they do, however, we see a lover who is attentive, devoted, and kind—if a bit moody. Venus in Cancer lovers are sensitive and prone to getting their feelings hurt easily! And they aren't quick to forget it, either. Regardless, though, a Cancer Venus will take their own fiercely protective nature and apply that to their loved ones. You can count on your Cancer babe to stand up for you and fight on your behalf if necessary.

Certainly we also see someone looking for commitment here. Similar to Venus in Taurus, Venus in Cancer loves a bit of predictability in their relationships. Knowing what to expect from their partners cultivates the security they crave, and they're happy as hell to settle into a routine early on. A solid, reliable partner and connection is the key to a Cancer Venus's heart. Even the most mature of them will be nervous about being left high and dry, so it's difficult to overstate the importance of safety, trust, and security here.

At the end of the day, family-oriented Venus in Cancer is looking for someone they can build with. A short-lived fling or anything of a casual nature just isn't that appealing to them. This isn't to say they don't end up with experiences of that sort—we all know how dating goes—but their preference is for someone who is serious and shares the same values.

Beyond this, Venus in Cancer is looking for a lot of snuggling, sweetness, and sentimentality. Anything too harsh or brash will leave these lovers feeling cold and turned off. Love interests who lack compassion and emotional depth will get left in the dust, as will anybody who doesn't make them feel cared for.

Keys to Empowerment

With Venus in Cancer, more than anything else it's important to own your values around family, commitment, and the need to feel safe and secure in your relationships. Whether people voice it or not, all of us are looking for a partner who helps us feel confident about their feelings for us. We all want to feel like we can rely on our partners to be there for us and know that we can trust them to treat us well, to be honest and loyal and kind. For a Cancer Venus, it is, in fact, a necessity, so there's no reason to feel shame around knowing that about yourself. Owning it will actually help you to attract better partners and start to have the kinds of experiences you need in love.

With your Venus in Cancer, owning your need for affection, sweetness, and someone who is going to take care of you is crucial, too. You bring all these things to the table yourself, so why settle for anything less? Why subject yourself to a partner who doesn't share those same values and love languages?

It's okay to want the traditional things, like building a family and making a home together, even in a world full of hookups where it can feel like nobody wants those things anymore. Your sensitive heart isn't built for casualness, and trying to force it to morph into something that is fundamentally against its nature will only leave you feeling hollow and resentful.

VENUS IN LEO

As astrology's golden child, Venus in Leo is magnetic AF. Leo is often associated with royalty, and Venus takes on a certain refinement and confidence here, exuding an aura that is, you guessed it, regal.

With Venus in the sign of the cosmic lion, these lovers are charismatic and full of joy and life and possess a warm, burning heart. They are proud and warmhearted and love to court and be courted. In astrology, Leo rules over the heart (and the hair!), so it's no surprise that Venus fares well here, able to blend the Venusian ideals of love with the generosity, loyalty, and playfulness of Leo.

It's true that Venus in Leo lovers need a lot of attention. That's just the way it is. Leo has a strong need to be acknowledged for the things that set them apart from the crowd, and Venus here is no exception. A Leo Venus will always need to be unique and exceptional and therefore require a partner who recognizes these qualities in them and will name them out loud. Flattery will get you everywhere with these lovers, and you can rest assured they will return the favor. Leo is actually quite boastful in love: They love to show off their partners and be shown off right back.

Loyalty is the name of the game for a Leo Venus, so they're typically not the type to stray. Remember that love is the most important thing for them. However, these lovers do thrive on romantic attention and may be a little *too* eager to share when someone has made a pass at them, if only because seeing a little bit of jealousy from their partner makes them feel all the more desired and special. Keep in mind that as much as they may love to dish out that kind of behavior, when the tables are turned, they won't see it as harmless—in fact, you'll see just how jealous and territorial they can be.

Another thing to remember is that Venus in Leo has high standards. These lovers expect a certain lifestyle and won't settle for anyone who can't give it to them or meet them at their level. They are ultimately looking to build an empire and truly need someone who can keep up and will work hard to create that kingdom together. However, remember that a Leo Venus can also be a lot of fun, and they value fun and joy in their connections.

Because Leo is the sign that rules over sex, physical affection is a big deal to them. Lovers with Venus in Leo have a strong sex drive and need a partner who can feed their appetite. Their need for love is arguably just as strong, so they can have difficulty separating love from sex. In their mind, the two are one in the same, and they may struggle with not equating sex with love. Venus in Leo is prone to having lots of sexual fantasies, but even those are often infused with love and affection. Though these individuals aren't likely to last long in sex-only connections, a loving relationship without the sexual component to match it will ultimately leave them unsatisfied and unhappy.

Keys to Empowerment

In my experience, those with Venus in Leo tend to feel a bit embarrassed about their need to feel special. However, when thinking about how to approach love and sex from a place of empowerment, it's important that you own this part of yourself. The truth is we *all* want to feel that way. And isn't one of the biggest joys of being in love the fact that you've found that special person who also thinks you're the greatest thing in the world? Pretending this isn't a need of yours is to deny who you truly are and what you truly desire. It will smother that warm, passionate, burning heart of yours, and in the end will extinguish the relationship. Leos are known for being bold and unapologetic about who they are. This same energy is what you need to bring to your love life, too.

With Venus in Leo, you will eventually have to confront your need for sex. Again, more often than not, this is a big issue in romantic relationships. Especially because love and sex go hand in hand for you, there's really no point in pretending otherwise. You need a partner who has a high sex drive, period, or at least one who is great in bed whenever you do connect that way.

Owning this desire—and perhaps downright need—is the only way to get what you want.

The only caveat is the need to be careful not to seek validation solely through sex. This is actually quite common for Leo placements, but it isn't necessarily healthy. With your Leo Venus, what other ways can you receive that validation in relationships that have nothing to do with the physical? How can you give that validation to yourself?

VENUS IN VIRGO

In the sign of the Virgin, Venus is said to be in its fall. Similar to when a planet is in detriment, there is something about the nature of a sign in its fall—in this case, Virgo—that feels fundamentally different from the natural qualities of the planet. This leaves the planet feeling ill at ease, and it may struggle to manifest in a way that feels good. However, as somebody who has lots of placements in both fall and detriment in my own chart, I tend to think this is a matter of perspective. For example, Virgo is the sign of service and devotion, both qualities that are beautiful and important to have when it comes to love. That said, many of the Virgo lovers I know have expressed their struggles when it comes to understanding how to make a relationship work. Let's talk about it.

As the second of the three earth signs, Virgo is extremely practical. Thanks to Mercury, its ruling planet, Virgo has a meticulous eye for detail and is highly analytical in nature. Thanks to their discerning eye, these lovers have high standards, both of others and of themselves. For better or worse, this desire to make everything (including their relationships) as good as possible tends to come off (and come out) a bit critical. Those with Venus in Virgo are direct as hell in their communication. They really aren't ones to beat around the bush or mince words, and they don't tend to sugarcoat their words. The hard part, in my opinion, is that a Virgo Venus truly is just trying to help. Their intentions are genuine and their hearts are true, and it is *because* of this that a tricky dynamic tends to arise in their relationships. On the one hand, I do think it's important that anybody involved with a Venus in Virgo lover recognizes that they are truly just trying to make things easier or better in some way. On the other hand, however, Virgo needs to understand that people generally don't like to be criticized, and even though their intentions are good, it doesn't negate the real impact of their words.

Now, there are plenty of ways to handle this. At the end of the day, those with Venus in Virgo will probably do best with someone who doesn't take their criticisms personally. Someone who is less sensitive and more practical (like them) may be a better fit. However, as communication is an imperative part of maintaining relationships of all kinds, there are some important lessons for these lovers around delivery.

The flip side of this is that because acts of service are the hallmark of Venus in Virgo, these lovers are very busy trying to make things work. They spend a lot of energy in the day-to-day trying to take care of things to ensure that everything in the relationship is running smoothly. The hard part for them is they often do it so quietly that much of their efforts go unnoticed! And there's nothing that hurts a Virgo Venus more than not feeling appreciated for their innumerable efforts. Thus, it is crucial that they find themselves a lover who recognizes all they do and consistently voices their appreciation for them. Honestly, once those with Venus in Virgo feel acknowledged this way, they are pretty low-maintenance partners.

Keys to Empowerment

Without a doubt, the most important thing for you to do as a Venus in Virgo lover is to find yourself a partner who actually sees and appreciates all the little things you do for them each day and will also *voice* that appreciation. While you may not show your love for someone with more stereotypical grand displays of affection, that doesn't make the way you love any less valid or powerful. You bring a lot to the table, and it's okay to know that! At the end of the day, feeling unappreciated and unacknowledged for all you do for your partner is the kiss of death, especially since once this need is met, you're a pretty low-maintenance partner.

With your Venus in Virgo, communication in general is key. The general approach you take is being willing to talk pretty much everything out. You're smart, and having a partner who is equally smart and values communication as much as you do is an absolute must. It's also important that they have their shit together.

That's right, Venus in Virgo—I know you have a tendency to take on people like projects, but in the long run that isn't sustainable. Everyone needs help sometimes, and it's good to be there for the people you care about, but not when you always have to help them. You're so very competent—imagine what you could do in a relationship with someone who matches your competency.

VENUS IN LIBRA

Venus finds its home in the sign of the scales, taking up its second domicile in the palace of Lady Justice. In Libra, the sign of partnership, Venus finds an ease of expression that we only see in two other places: Taurus and Pisces.

The main thing to understand about Venus in Libra lovers is that they love love. They are happiest when they're in a partnership, and they take a kind, balanced, evenhanded approach to love. Because they innately understand that relationships require both give and take, compromise is their specialty. In fact, their default setting is to prioritize the other person. They can be quite focused on their partners, always wanting to know how they're doing, what they're thinking, and what they want and need. They are more likely to give in to their partner's wants, ultimately looking to maintain the peace, which they value oh so very much.

There is a polished nature that Venus in Libra naturally embodies as well. They are the grace of Venus incarnate and want to look, feel, and be lovely. Because of this, these lovers are turned off by anything harsh, rude, or distasteful. To some this may come off as a bit shallow or superficial, but really, Libra is a gentle sign that has a strong aversion to bad manners or any kind of cruelty. Therefore, it's very important for those with Venus here to have gentle partners, as it's too easy for them to get bullied or pushed around by more aggressive ones.

Certainly, these lovers are charming beyond measure. Their Venusian grace extends to their personalities, generally making them attractive not only physically but also through the way they conduct themselves with others.

Venus in Libra can be a shameless flirt! These lovers are never short on potential love interests, which can be both a beautiful and a dangerous thing. If we're being honest, sometimes Venus in Libra loves the idea of love rather than the actual practice of it. These babes idealize love, and it can be a harsh lesson when reality doesn't match up with their vision. When that happens, they can be quick to flee the scene and jump right into another relationship with whoever is next in line.

When they do find someone to stick with, those with Venus in Libra treat their partners with unwavering fairness. They treat their partners well, with kindness and a willingness to see the other side.

Keys to Empowerment

I think the most empowering thing a Venus in Libra can do is accept their desire for a relationship. In a world that thrives on hookups and being perpetually single, desiring a real connection can be hard. However, the very nature of Libra is to be in a partnership, and to deny this part of yourself would be to stifle your true essence.

However, with your Venus in Libra, keep in mind that as you strive for true balance and equality in your relationships, part of that balance requires that you learn to place just as much value on your own wants and needs as you do on the other person's. The natural state of Libra is to give, give, give, and there are plenty of lessons here around learning to receive, too, especially because you usually *do* know what you want! You don't always have to compromise to keep the peace. True equality comes from giving your partner the opportunity to compromise, too, and the opportunity to do what *you* want to do for once. You might be surprised at just how willing your partner is to give you that same care and consideration in return.

Speaking of learning to let it be about you for once, there is a journey for all Libra placements around autonomy. Especially with Venus here, these lovers can be a bit codependent, placing much of their self-worth in their relationship status and/or needing other people to define who they are in some way. With your Venus in Libra, learning to stand on your own without the constant need for others to reflect back who you are, even when in a relationship, is super important. And in that sense, having strong boundaries is important, too, as it will help you maintain the distance you need to have clarity.

VENUS IN SCORPIO

In Scorpio, Venus finds itself in the second sign of its detriment. Similar to Aries, Scorpio is traditionally ruled by Mars, lending itself to a sharper, darker energy that Venus struggles to thrive in. That said, this is arguably the most passionate position of Venus.

Venus in Scorpio lovers are deep, dark, and passionate creatures, full of intensity, ardor, and desire. They possess a highly magnetic aura that is also a bit mysterious, giving them a healthy dose of allure that draws others to them. Something about their energy can be a bit provocative, thick with a sultry, seductive promise.

The most important thing to understand about a Scorpio Venus is they're not looking for anything causal. These lovers are looking to merge bodies, minds, hearts, and souls, and will settle for nothing less. Because of this, it takes a long time for someone to actually catch the eye of a Scorpio Venus, let alone catch their attention in any serious way. But once someone does manage to snare their attention, it's on like Donkey Kong.

A Venus in Scorpio lover is going to give you their full attention. They're highly focused on their partners, and something about the way they move communicates the promise of fierce loyalty, deep commitment, and sexual pleasure—though it's unlikely they'd ever tell you this directly. As with all Scorpio placements, Scorpio Venus lovers are private and guarded, especially in the beginning. They will want to explore all your nooks and crannies and hear your secrets, seeking to know every single inch of who you are, but don't expect them to be forthcoming with their own. It takes a long time for these lovers to open up.

The closed-off nature of a Scorpio Venus is a result of them having undergone some seriously painful experiences in love. Things like lies, betrayal, cheating, and so on are unfortunately quite common for those with this Venus placement. Romantic relationships are the battleground for transformation in a way that isn't true for everyone else. The pain of betrayal in love cuts bone-deep, and it takes them a long time to move on—sometimes years and years. Because of this, Venus in Scorpio lovers are guarded with their heart and definitely struggle with trust, hence it takes them a while to feel safe enough to open up and share again. Much patience and understanding will be required of their love interests and partners. Still, the full attention of these lovers can be seductive, as they somehow make it seem attractive to be possessed by them.

It's true that a Scorpio Venus can be a little toxic in this way—jealousy and possessiveness are all too common here. Depending on your personality, these traits can be sexy as hell or totally repulsive. Regardless, their full-body commitment commands the same energy from their partners, and they won't tolerate any kind of shady behavior. Mutual obsession is the only acceptable option, and gaining the trust of these lovers requires showing your full commitment to them. Venus in Scorpio isn't afraid of intimacy, so you better not be, either.

Speaking of intimacy, sex is a big deal to a Scorpio Venus. Thanks to their Martian nature, these lovers are highly sexual. They have a voracious sex drive and look to express their impossibly strong ardor physically. Similar to what we saw with Venus in Leo, sex may in fact be a downright need for Venus in Scorpio, and if their partner can't match their level of desire, they will wilt on the vine.

Keys to Empowerment

Above all else, the key to empowerment for Venus in Scorpio lies in owning your intensity and passion. While others may shy away from your intensity or have trouble handling it, it honestly doesn't matter. I know you've likely had experiences that left you feeling like no one seems to feel as deeply or as passionately as you do, but I promise they're out there. It's difficult to overstate the importance of finding a lover who can match your depth and level of ardor—without it, you'll never be satisfied. Therefore, anybody who isn't as serious as you or doesn't crave the all-encompassing connection you desire would ultimately be unfulfilling anyway. At the end of the day, you're looking for mutual obsession. Why torture yourself with someone who is incapable of giving you what you need?

The other necessity for a Scorpio Venus is finding acceptance around the fact that it will probably take you longer to find lovers and enter into relationships. Again, because you're hunting for something very special, you probably won't get involved in as many relationships or flings as those around you. That's okay. The wait will be worth it in the end.

Finally, because relationships are the stage of transformation for Venus in Scorpio, at some point you're going to have to do the work to stop learning from the deeply painful sides of love and instead learn from its healing, healthy qualities. Don't forget that there's something about the way *you* love that is deeply transforming for others as well. We have to show up ready to offer the healing gifts of love, too.

VENUS IN SAGITTARIUS

Venus in Sagittarius, which has a reputation for being one of the forever single signs, is difficult to pin down, generally speaking.

In jubilant, jovial Sagittarius, Venus leaves behind the intensity of Scorpio for a life full of laughter, independence, and lightheartedness, and these lovers are looking for someone who is the same. Venus in Sagittarius isn't one for super heavy or super emo connections at all. On the contrary, these lovers are ready to flee the scene if things feel too overdone or restrictive. They're ultimately looking for somebody to experience the adventure of life with and will wilt in a relationship with a homebody or a controlling, negative Nancy.

Those with a Sagittarius Venus are ready to strike out into the world and have all kinds of experiences when it comes to love and partnerships. They may seek to connect with all kinds of different people and have just as many varying experiences when it comes to sex and romance. They learn best through firsthand experience, and in this case it's the experience of relationships. Through these diverse encounters they are able to further develop their personal philosophy on love. Because of Sagittarius's connection to foreign lands and cultures, this position of Venus can indicate someone who prefers to date people from different cultural backgrounds.

Keep in mind that Venus in Sagittarius is optimistic and full of life! These lovers are open to embracing the beauty of love in all its facets and allowing it to expand their horizons. The heart—just like the mind—works best when it's open. At the end of the day, if these lovers don't feel they can grow within or because of a relationship, they will put it to bed. This isn't to say that Venus in Sagittarius is incapable of commitment, though. Once they find someone who shares their beliefs and values, they go all in. In fact, they can be a somewhat confusing mix of serious and casual, as even when they are in a committed relationship things always need to remain a bit light. Humor, witty banter, and laughter are the pillars of any good relationship where Venus in Sagittarius is concerned. If you can make them laugh, you've snared their attention, and the two of you will crack up all the way to the bedroom.

Thanks to their fiery nature, Venus in Sagittarius babes are blunt AF in their approach. If they like you, you'll know it, as they have no qualms about voicing their interest and asking someone out. Be careful, though! If you aren't into it or are wishy-washy in any way, they're just as fast to leave you in the dust and move on to something and someone else. At the end of the day, you don't need to be polished or refined to attract a Sagittarius Venus, but you better be prepared to engage in deep, philosophical conversations and show your appreciation of their views.

Keys to Empowerment

With Venus in Sagittarius, the most important thing you can do for yourself is own your joie de vivre. Life is, in fact, the most wonderful and beautiful thing, and wanting to see and experience as much of it as you can is the right approach. Furthermore, empowerment comes through owning your desire to experience all of it with someone.

With your Venus in Sagittarius, you will never be satisfied with someone who doesn't share this same perspective and/or wants to stay at home. Finding someone who shares your zest for life and wants to strike out into the world and explore with you is the only thing that will satiate you, and there's no point in engaging with someone who is going to weigh you down or try to smother your big heart and big dreams. Freedom and independence are your bread and butter, and you need a partner who values those things, too, and will give them to you in great swaths. Don't feel bad about moving on quickly from someone if and when it becomes clear that your values don't align. Just make sure you're honest about it.

As you travel the world, stay open to the idea of meeting someone while you're abroad. It might just be the greatest thing a Venus in Sagittarius can do.

VENUS IN CAPRICORN

Generally speaking, Venus in Capricorn lovers are the most traditional of the bunch. As the sign that rules over things like the government and the powers that be, and the systems and structures we need in place to maintain them, perhaps it's no surprise that this Venus placement trends toward the old guard. They hold traditional values in high regard—likely stemming from whatever values were instilled in them by their parents—and in that same vein, they possess a sense of duty or responsibility toward their partners and partnerships.

Like everything else in their lives, Venus in Capricorn lovers have a vision when it comes to romance. They are playing the long game and know what it is they're looking to build with someone. Because of this, the name of the game for these lovers is commitment. They take that word seriously, and if they feel they can't take someone else seriously, they won't waste their time. More than anything else, a Capricorn Venus lives in their integrity, and they value integrity when it comes to love. They will unwaveringly embody their values and will expect the same from a partner. Anything less is unacceptable.

Keep in mind, too, that these individuals are nothing if not practical, and they don't allow their emotions to cloud their vision. If you don't share the same long-term goals and values or you act in ways that they view as flaky or uncouth, Venus in Capricorn won't be calling you again.

The flip side of this is that a Capricorn Venus loves to take care of their partners, and they do so in the quintessential earth sign way: through the practical and tangible. This sign is the astrological sugar daddy—they will buy you nice, albeit probably useful, things and naturally take on the dominant role of tending to bills, etc. (or at least the evolved, mature ones will).

One thing I really want to drive home here is that just because Venus in Capricorn trends toward logic doesn't mean they are unfeeling. The symbol of this sign is the sea goat: half-goat, half-fish. Yes, Capricorn is an earth sign, but alongside their grounded, reserved nature is a highly developed intuition. Those with Venus in Capricorn know exactly how they feel, but they aren't ones for grand gestures or public displays. These lovers are private, and it isn't until you're alone, away from the masses, that they will tell you how they feel. They'd rather be alone together anyway.

Keys to Empowerment

With Venus in Capricorn, own the fact that you're a serious person looking for a serious relationship. There's no use in pretending otherwise. It's a beautiful thing to be crystal clear about what you're looking for in a partner and a long-term relationship, something that evades most people until they're older. Remaining true to yourself and your standards is the only thing that's going to make you happy, so why lower your standards and settle? It's okay to wait until you find someone you can take seriously and to be ruthlessly discerning until you do. In today's modern age, where dating involves a lot of swiping and ghosting, you'll only frustrate yourself trying to stoop down to behavior that doesn't align with your values. As a person who lives in their integrity and approaches love honestly, you are a much-needed breath of fresh air.

It's also important to get comfortable with valuing more traditional norms in love, which is the true nature of Venus in Capricorn, after all. Trying to push yourself to fit into a mold that goes fundamentally against what you desire in order to fit in with modern dating will only leave you feeling bitter and resentful. Monogamy is beautiful, too. Wanting to take care of your partner, wanting to build something substantial over the long term, wanting to buy a house and maybe have some kids—you understand what it means to truly walk the path of life with someone. Own it. Be up-front about it. You're worth it.

VENUS IN AQUARIUS

The planet of love puts on its most eclectic mask in the electric field of quixotic Aquarius. Like all planets in the water bearer's domain, there is something unconventional about Venus here.

In Aquarius, Venus breaks free from the traditional ideals of Capricorn and approaches relationships from a different space. First we see more of an emphasis on friendship, or at the very least Venus in Aquarius teaches us the value of having a solid foundation of friendship built into our romantic connections. It's important to *like* our partners, not just love them. Very often this placement is where we see the friends-to-lovers trope play out in real life. We also tend to see things like polyamory, ethical nonmonogamy, and any and all versions of relationships that are experimental and outside of the norm.

Of course, this isn't *always* the case. Sometimes Venus in Aquarius is simply someone who is attracted to strong individuals and people who may seem outside the box in some way. Aquarius is able to see the beauty in all walks of life and appreciates people for who they truly are. It's our quirks that Aquarius loves the most. These individuals are more apt than any other Venus placement to accept their lovers exactly as they are.

It's important to understand that Venus in Aquarius values freedom in relationships. In fact, for them, this is arguably the most important component of any connection. These lovers are extremely independent and tend to be a bit aloof, valuing (and requiring!) space above all else, even with those they're head over heels for. Clinginess, at least in the beginning, tends to be the kiss of death for them. Keep in mind also that Venus in Aquarius tends to be most attracted to people when *they* are aloof or unreachable in some way, as maddening as that may be. This Venus placement is a bit of an enigma. However, once they're interested, they can become fixated—Aquarius is a fixed sign, after all.

Keys to Empowerment

With Venus in Aquarius, it's difficult to overstate the importance of owning who you are and what you believe when it comes to relationships. One of the hardest things for Aquarius placements is that the road tends to be quite lonely. As the futurists of the zodiac—often living on the bleeding edge of all things—they tend to experience a life full of people not truly understanding their vision or perspective. Those with Venus in Aquarius are early adopters of all things, and relationships are no exception. In that sense, other people may not quite understand their values or approach to things, like marriage, for example. It doesn't really matter, though, as there will always be a small few who do, and they will be *obsessed*. Wait for them.

With Venus in Aquarius, it's so important to own your need for space and freedom. In my experience, these lovers truly need a partner who isn't threatened by their need for alone time. After you go out into the ether and explore whatever it is you wish to explore, you need a partner who will be waiting for you with open arms when you return. There is safety in that, and finding or cultivating that dynamic in your partnerships will help it—and you—thrive.

VENUS IN PISCES

It is here, in the final sign of the zodiac, that we find Venus in her exaltation. A planet is exalted whenever it's in a sign that shares many of the same characteristics and motivations as that planet. This brings a palpable ease to the planet, making it feel good and giving it a certain power that is similar to when the planet is in domicile. In that sense, Venus loves to be in Pisces.

This last sign in the zodiacal wheel is mutable water, bringing a healthy dose of flexibility, understanding, and tender emotions to the sign of the fishes. Venus in Pisces is deeply sensitive and empathetic, with a soft, kind heart. These lovers are able to see the beauty in each and every one of us, regardless of background, age, creed, or anything. Thanks to this gift, of all the signs in the zodiac, Pisces embodies the ideal of unconditional love in a real way that the rest of us could stand to learn from.

The ability to see the good in everyone gives Venus in Pisces lovers a bit of an indiscriminate taste. Similar to when Venus is in Aquarius, it may seem like there's no rhyme or reason to their choice in mates, and sometimes their choices may even be a bit confusing or shocking to those around them. No matter who they link up with, though, a Venus in Pisces lover will want to spend a lot of time with their love. Indeed, they are happiest when they can spend as much time as possible with their partner, even if it's simply joining them in a car ride to the gas station. For these lovers, there is no such thing as too much time together or being too close.

This desire to merge with their partner stems from the inherent boundlessness of this sign. Those with Venus in Pisces are locked in a dreamworld, with a predisposition toward fantasy and romance that they are ready to project onto any and every one of their lovers. Not to take the wind out of your sails, Venus in Pisces, but if this is you, it's important that you are able to really see your partner for who they really are and the relationship for what it really is, rather than ignoring real issues and choosing to see things the way you'd like them to be.

Because Venus in Pisces tends to only see the good in others, and perhaps has weaved a fantasy around others, boundaries are of the utmost importance. In my experience, most Pisces placements usually go through some harsh reality checks as they learn that not everyone possesses the same kind heart that they do. Unfortunately, the kindness of Venus in Pisces can have these lovers getting taken advantage of by those who wish to exploit their goodwill for personal gain. Now, this isn't to discourage these lovers from embodying their true nature, but simply to say that discernment is key. There are still those out there who deserve all their loving kindness!

Keys to Empowerment

With Venus in Pisces, it's extremely important that you confront the idea of sacrifice when it comes to love. Very often you may feel that the two are one in the same—and while we do have to make sacrifices for the ones we love *sometimes*, this shouldn't be a dynamic that exists *always*. Establishing boundaries is one of the most important things for Pisces placements, and being able to say no and stand up for yourself will change the dynamic in your connections in a healthy way. Learning that you don't have to give all parts of yourself in order to receive love will fundamentally change your relationship dynamics as well.

That said, I do believe that part of empowerment for a Pisces Venus involves owning your soft, romantic side. It's perfectly okay to love love and to love being in love. As I mentioned above, these individuals truly embody the idea of unconditional love, and I think the most empowering thing a Pisces Venus can do is lead by example. Teach the rest of us the power of having an open heart in a world that so often wants us to close it off.

A NOTE ON THE HOUSES

When looking at the house Venus sits in, we gain another layer of nuance and understanding about our approach to love, beauty, pleasure, and romance. There are several factors that play into Venus's influence in a house, which can be quite complex.

First, we can see where Venus bestows us with its charm, beauty, and grace. For example, someone with Venus in the first house naturally embodies their Venusian energy, and these lovers are often considered quite attractive and charming by others. Someone with Venus in their fourth house is likely to have a beautiful home.

Next, we can see where and how we channel or express our Venusian energy, as well as how we like love to show up in our lives. Venus in the sixth house denotes someone who wants to have their partner(s) be a part of their everyday lives. Once in a relationship, these lovers will work to make seeing their love interest a part of their daily routine. They may also need a certain amount of general enjoyment and pleasure woven into their day-to-day lives, whereas lovers with Venus in the twelfth house struggle greatly to access and express all their Venusian faculties. This doesn't mean there isn't plenty of love to give, however! It's simply that Venus twelfth housers tend to need more time to feel comfortable opening up and expressing all they have to give. Having a partner (or partners!) who understand this about them is crucial.

The final thing to note about the house containing Venus is it can also show the qualities we value in life and relationships, as well as the type of partner or partners we're looking for and how we might meet them. Personally I think the best two examples of this are Venus in the ninth house and the eleventh house. When Venus is in the ninth house, the person may meet someone while traveling or in college, and/or they may be more attracted to people from different cultures than their own. For someone with Venus in the eleventh house, the best way to meet someone is through people they already know. Maybe the love of their life is a friend of a friend, or they meet them at a barbecue at their neighbor's house, or perhaps they even meet them online, as the eleventh house also rules over social media. Really understanding the nature of the house your Venus lives in can help you have an easier time getting your love life off and popping.

The fifth house is the house of joy for Venus in astrology. Hellenistic astrology gives this house the title "the House of Good Fortune." Again, as the house of joy, pleasure, and romance, the fifth house has a lot in common with Venus. Because the fifth house is also about children and our inner child, those with Venus here may have been quite young when their interest in love first emerged. They may have started dating quite young as well. This is one indication of someone who loves love and is focused on romance. At the very least, these lovers seem to always have a crush.

Certainly, people with Venus in the fifth house experience a great deal of fun and pleasure in their lives. There is a natural ease around these themes, and they want to enjoy all that life has to offer to its fullest extent. Art and beauty surround these folks, and they're likely sensual and creative by nature. They are warm, playful, charming, and easily charmed.

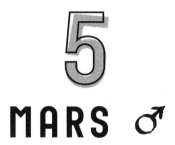

MARS ♂

DOMICILE: Aries and Scorpio

EXALTATION: Capricorn

DETRIMENT: Libra and Taurus

FALL: Cancer

In astrology, Mars is the other etheric lover, the perfect counterpart to Venus, and makes up the other half of the partnership planets. As the planet of sex, Mars is the most obvious placement to study when it comes to sextrology. The sign Mars sits in perhaps best represents our sexual style in its rawest form. This is where we will first look into potential turn-ons and turnoffs, as well as how we approach sex in general. The position of Mars in the chart points to our wants, needs, and desires; it is our sexual appetite. Because of Mars's association with drive, it also points to the hunt: How do we pursue these desires? How do we go after sex? How do we view sex? As a conquest? As a soul-bonding experience?

Sharing its namesake with the god of war, Mars represents the masculine principle—which is to say our active side. Beyond just sex, Mars symbolizes passion in all its varying manifestations. It is the planet of vitality, assertion, action, boundaries, conflict, and anger, which are also important—and inevitable—aspects of relationships. The sign that Mars sits in also represents how we show up in conflict, how our anger expresses itself, and how and where we direct that energy. Everything about Mars is physical, visceral. Any

♂

THE POSITION OF MARS IN THE CHART POINTS TO OUR WANTS, NEEDS, AND DESIRES. IT DESCRIBES OUR SEXUAL APPETITE AND OUR POTENTIAL TURN-ONS AND TURNOFFS.

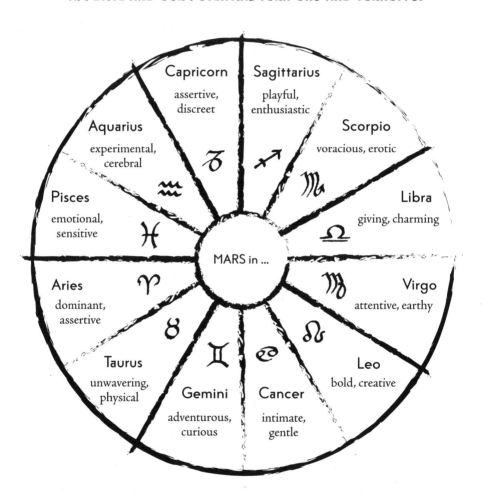

Capricorn
assertive, discreet

Sagittarius
playful, enthusiastic

Scorpio
voracious, erotic

Aquarius
experimental, cerebral

Libra
giving, charming

Pisces
emotional, sensitive

MARS in ...

Virgo
attentive, earthy

Aries
dominant, assertive

Leo
bold, creative

Taurus
unwavering, physical

Gemini
adventurous, curious

Cancer
intimate, gentle

and every Martian characteristic manifests through the body, one way or another.

Mars is both how we fuck and fight.

As is the case with Venus, there is plenty to glean from learning about both your own Mars and your loved one's.

MARS IN ARIES

We kick off our journey with Mars in its home sign of Aries. As the ruling planet of the first sign of the zodiac, Mars is powerfully placed and operates at peak performance here.

Those with their Mars in Aries burn *hot*, especially in the bedroom. Aries is all about the chase, the hunt, the pursuit, and tends to get off on it. This is especially true if they feel their partner is giving themselves over in a way that feels pure or innocent—the opposite of their powerful, dominating sexual prowess. In fact, for these lovers there's something about asserting their physical power that is innately tied to getting off. Nothing about an Aries Mars is passive; in fact, they're likely to be turned off by a partner who tries to overpower their dominant nature or is too assertive. They want to be the one to do the pursuing, period.

If a Mars in Aries wants you, you'll know it, likely because they've straight up told you. These lovers thrive in the heat of the moment, wanting sex to be spontaneous, fresh, and new. Certainly they don't want to overthink anything, as that can be a mood killer. Plus, in true Aries fashion, they're impatient lovers. Too much foreplay only impedes their desire to get, well, straight to the point. Aries lovers are extremely passionate, and especially through the lens of Mars, they have a lot of energy to burn. They're like a Little Caesars pizza: hot and ready.

It's true that these lovers can be a bit selfish in bed, as is the Aries way, but as they mature over time, they learn the value of giving in bed, if only because it's another way for them to hone, sharpen, and show off their awesome sexual skills.

As Aries rules over the head, it's actually an erogenous zone for these lovers! They love when their partner runs their fingers through their hair or messes it up or grabs their face. Because of the quick-moving nature of Mars in Aries, these people are quick to get fired up, love a good quickie, and are just as fast to move on. They are sincere and passionate in their sexual expression though not necessarily constant. Again, it largely depends on the moment.

As far as conflict is concerned, you'll know exactly where you stand with Mars in Aries. These lovers are bold and courageous as hell and are unlikely to back down from a fight. Their anger can be explosive and powerful, seeming to rise almost out of thin air. And then, once that anger has been expressed, it leaves just as quickly as it flared up. These folks are easily irritated by indirectness from others, as they themselves are as direct as can be. Similar to their approach to sexuality, they are sincere in their expression of anger, and you can trust they don't have a hidden agenda.

MARS IN TAURUS

In Venus-ruled Taurus, Mars takes on a much different form than in Aries. Mars is in its detriment here, as the warrior planet struggles to assert itself the way it wants to under the soft Venusian influence. However, just as we've seen with Venus in detriment (in both Scorpio and Aries), having your Mars in Taurus is no reason to fret. Remember that in antiquity, Venus was also the goddess of war, and she has plenty to offer in the bullpen.

When Mars is in detriment, it's believed that the planet struggles to express itself in an effective way. This is largely due to the fact that Taurus is an incredibly slow-moving sign, so it struggles to get started. However, once it does, there's no stopping it.

Taurus also brings its Venusian sensuality to the sexual potency of Mars, giving these lovers a very hands-on, physical expression of sex, as well as incredible stamina. These are the people who can truly go all night long. In that sense, their sexual appetite gets a voracious boost that may feel difficult to satiate. Anything and everything that stimulates the physical senses is erotic for Mars in Taurus: touch, smell, taste. While they may not be very spontaneous, preferring a steady approach to sex, they are quite good at what they do. Because of their gluttonous sexual appetite, abstinence is especially difficult for them, and they do best with a constant, regular sexual partner.

Though these lovers are slow to anger, even in detriment that anger has to come out somehow. When finally pushed past their breaking point, a Taurus Mars is like a bulldozer: They will plow through and over anything and everything, including you. They can be quite domineering in this way, and thanks to their bull-like stubbornness, you're probably not going to talk them out of it. In that sense, we also see someone who is probably going to hold a grudge. That's one of Taurus's superpowers, after all. That anger built up over a long period of time, and it's going to take just as long, if not longer, for it to leave. Good luck.

MARS IN GEMINI

In Gemini, Mars takes on a much busier energy than in Taurus. Because Gemini is interested in so many different things, Mars here seeks to direct itself through a bunch of different avenues, which is to say these lovers have a lot going on. These are likely people who are always on the move, seeking to put thought into action, and who have a great need to have outlets for their buzzing energy. In that sense, they may be a bit restless and get bored easily, needing constant action to feel adequately stimulated.

This same need extends to the bedroom. Mars in Gemini lovers prefer variety both in partners and in sexual contact. They can be quite adventurous, curious lovers who are down to do it in any position you're willing to try! Oral pleasure is their specialty, and they love, love, love to kiss.

Mars in Gemini is the lover you can talk dirty to, and you can be certain they'll give it right back. The main aphrodisiac for these busy lovers is conversation and an intellectual connection in general—foreplay begins outside the bedroom in that sense. They are driven more through the intellect than through their desires. They can be quite vocal once you do get them in the bedroom, however, and they're going to want to hear you scream.

When Mars in Gemini lovers express anger, their words cut like a knife. When provoked, their tongues are sharp and their words become their weapon. They can be quite sarcastic and condescending, though in true Gemini fashion they'll change their mind quickly and move on once they've been able to voice their anger. These lovers do best with someone they can vent their frustrations to, as they ultimately just need to get things off their chest.

MARS IN CANCER

Here in the first of the three water signs of the zodiac, Mars is in its fall. As with any other planet in the sign of its fall, we see a certain tension between the characteristics and desires of Cancer and those of Mars, the planet of action, conflict, and sex. By nature, Mars loves to be out and moving in the world. The god of war thrives on bold actions and the heat of the moment, but Cancer, in stark contrast, is self-protective and can be downright shy, preferring to observe and take its time feeling out people and situations. There is a fundamental need for safety in all things, which manifests as Cancer needing to determine whether they feel safe enough to open up, act, etc. Mars wants to go, go, go, but Cancer says wait, wait, wait.

We see this same apprehension extend to the bedroom. Unlike any of the other Mars placements covered thus far, Mars in Cancer truly needs the deep emotional intimacy they crave in order to have the most fulfilling sex. These are sensitive, sweet lovers who trend toward romance and whispering sweet nothings in your ear. Romantic, sensual touches add a little something extra for them, and they definitely want to cuddle afterward.

Certainly Mars in Cancer lovers are submissive. They need partners who are more aggressive and they may even like it when you're a little mean to them in bed—as long as they know you love them. The chest is an erogenous zone for them, and, yes, they love a good set of tits, where appropriate. They may also get turned on by the idea of making a baby—even if only in theory.

When thinking about Cancer through the Martian lens, we see the self-protective nature of the crab shine through. Like any other Cancer placement, a certain moodiness exists in a Cancer Mars. And once their feelings have been hurt, you're going to either be on the receiving end of their bone-crushing claws or have them pull away into their crabby shell, or both. There is a surprising stubbornness that exists with Mars in Cancer that rarely shows its face. Should they opt to escape into their shell to lick their wounds, there's no pulling them back out until they're good and ready. There's little to be done save for stepping away and letting them have their space and as much time as they need.

MARS IN LEO

In astrology, Leo is the sign that rules over sex. With Mars, the planet of sex, in the Leonine fires, there is a certain level of comfort and natural prowess. This is an especially vital position for Mars, full of passion and desire. The pride of the lion shines through the sexual lens, giving these lovers a stunning confidence in their sexual abilities, which motivates them to do their best in bed.

Thanks to their innate creativity, those with a Leo Mars are prone to lots of sexual fantasies. Due to the self-centered nature of the sign, many of their fantasies revolve around worship, obsession, and attention from their partners. Though they *will* make sure their partners are happy, they are truly most focused on their own pleasure. These lovers are easily aroused and enjoy sex more than most people. Their impressive sexual appetite means they do best with someone who can keep up and is down to fuck all the time.

As I mentioned in the Venus in Leo section, Mars in Leo has a difficult time untangling sex and love—the two may be conflated. Though these lovers are capable of having purely sexual relationships or situationships, they probably won't last that long, as Leo is going to get their feelings involved eventually and crave love and affection from their partner(s).

Thanks to their fiery nature, Mars in Leo lovers can come on quite strong. They are bold about who and what they want and can be quite jealous and possessive. They may even put their partners to a test, if only to see how much they truly desire them. Because of their extreme need for validation— and gratification!—they can get turned on by inequality during sex. Thanks to the fixed nature of Leo, these lovers have a lot of staying power.

While Mars in Cancer struggles to take action on pretty much anything, initiative returns with Mars in Leo. Be careful not to feed into any potential drama that gets drummed up from this tension—as is the Leo way! The easiest way to piss off a Mars in Leo lover is to humiliate them in some way or be disloyal in their eyes. Wounding their pride will send them roaring, and they will certainly bring the drama and passion into their expressions of anger. If you aren't looking to get mauled, get out of the way.

MARS IN VIRGO

Of all twelve positions of Mars, Virgo Mars lovers have the healthiest relationship with sex. They tend to view sex as a necessary function of a well-rounded approach to health and general well-being. They release everyday stress and tension through sex, whether with someone or by themselves. Both their sexual health and their partner's are very important to them.

Mars in Virgo lovers are most attracted to people who largely go unnoticed, preferring their lovers to be simple and sweet. They get revved up when they know their partner appreciates all the little things they do. In more extreme cases, they get turned on by the idea of being someone's (sexual) slave. Despite Virgo's reputation for perfectionism, Mars in this sign is the exact opposite. Instead, they are attracted to a person's imperfections and do best with partners who need or prefer lots of care.

In truth, Mars in Virgo babes may be rather inexperienced when it comes to sex, though they are insatiably curious about it. This inexperience can lend itself to insecurity that can only be overcome with time. Certainly they are givers in the bedroom, and they may even enjoy watching a bit. They definitely aim to please and want to "do well" in their lover's eyes.

It's important not to mistake Mars in Virgo's focus on health for a sign that they are vanilla. These lovers are *not* afraid to get down and dirty, especially within the confines of a committed relationship. In fact, once they feel comfortable with their partners, you may be surprised at just how nasty they can truly be!

Now, being on the receiving end of a Mars in Virgo's anger is actually awful. Similar to Mars in Gemini, a Virgo Mars will wield their words as a weapon, and the blow is devastating. This is thanks to the sharp, discerning, and analytical nature of Virgo. Their words drip with a venomous criticism that also happens to be correct, making their attacks especially calculated and lethal. Though they aren't quick to anger, you can trust that they've been categorizing all the things that have been annoying or pissing them off for a while, and their vitriol is backed up by dates, times, locations, receipts, and straight facts.

Oops.

MARS IN LIBRA

In Venus-ruled Libra, Mars is said to be in its detriment, just like when it's in Taurus. And it's true that Mars is a bit funny in the sign of the scales, especially when it comes to sex. These are the pickiest lovers around without a doubt! Because Libra values beauty and refinement, wanting everything to be of high quality and taste, those with a Libra Mars are uncharacteristically overt about what they do and don't like. This quality extends to sex as well. The mood, atmosphere, and style of lovemaking need to be just right.

Once a Mars in Libra lover does find a worthy partner, though, they aim to please. They are givers in bed to be sure, but trust that they expect you to give right back! Equality is the name of the game, after all, and they are looking for a balanced approach to giving and receiving.

Certainly Mars in Libra is quite charming, as is every Libra placement. Under the Martian influence, that charm can turn downright provocative, though in a more subtle, graceful way than you might expect. These lovers are seeking sexual growth and will not stay with someone who doesn't offer that potential.

Beyond this, Libra rules over the lower back and the butt! Thus, these babes love being spanked or grabbed and will likely dish out a fair share of their own gropes. Because this is an erogenous zone for them, you might be surprised at just what they're down to try with the back door.

Conflict is an issue that makes those with Mars in Libra feel uneasy. As lovers of peace, they have a strong aversion to strife in relationships. More than any other position of Mars, a Libra Mars may downright avoid conflict. There are lots of obvious lessons here for these lovers, as conflict is an inevitable and unavoidable part of relationships, and whether they like it or not, anger is a feeling they're going to experience. Remember that eventually it has to go *somewhere*.

Because Mars in Libra strives for peace—and because they are understanding creatures by nature—there is a tendency to just let things go. The trouble, of course, is that they aren't actually letting it go. Instead, the problem tends to build up over time until it reaches its boiling point and they explode. This can be shocking for the person on the receiving end, as they may not even be aware the problem exists! Meanwhile, the Mars in Libra lover has been aware of the issue for a long time—sometimes months or even years—and will feel exasperated by this response. Learning to speak up sooner and be more up-front about what is bothering them is key to dismantling this dynamic in their relationships.

MARS IN SCORPIO

The scorpion's lair is the second domain for Mars, though the planet takes on a much different shape in watery Scorpio. As with all Scorpio placements, Mars in Scorpio has an alluring, magnetic aura that promises an impossible amount of sexual depth and intensity. Eye contact is the name of the game for these lovers, as they possess an incredible amount of focus—a focus that they'll lock on whoever has caught their eye.

Because Mars is at home in Scorpio, we again see lovers with a voracious sexual appetite and a natural prowess that manifests as a high sex drive. Their erotic nature is actually quite complex and can vary greatly in expression depending on experience and self-awareness. One thing you can count on, though, is they want it—all the time. Similar to Venus in Scorpio, a Scorpio Mars has a fundamental need to channel their passion physically, which makes sex very important to them. They need a partner who can keep up and who can successfully stoke the flames of passion as well.

Mars in Scorpio lovers desire full-body pleasure and may be attracted to power dynamics and things others consider to be taboo, such as kink. They will do almost anything in bed as long as they've found the right partner. Mars in Scorpio is an especially provocative, vital placement that is also exceedingly private. These lovers do not kiss and tell and prefer if you don't either.

Keep in mind that Mars in Scorpio can use sex as a means of control. Sometimes these lovers are prone to long periods of abstinence, withholding sex until they feel they and/or their partner are deserving. However, when it's time, this placement of Mars is believed to have the strongest sexual stamina of them all.

Where conflict is concerned, the keyword for Mars in Scorpio is revenge, and they know it's a dish best served cold. Perhaps more than any other Scorpio placement (besides Venus), Mars in Scorpio is prone to jealousy, possessiveness, resentment, and bitterness. And a slighted Scorpio Mars lover is *not* a cute sight.

Being on the receiving end of a Mars in Scorpio's anger is a precarious place to find yourself. Typically, a Scorpio Mars won't attack unless provoked, but if their anger has been seething and writhing under the surface for some time, then once you've given them a reason to defend themselves, you better be prepared for what comes next. These lovers make a formidable opponent and an even worse enemy.

MARS IN SAGITTARIUS

For Mars in Sagittarius, sex is an adventure or a sport. The blunt, straightforward nature of the archer expresses itself readily through the lens of Mars, which enables these lovers to tell you directly when they're into you. They're also rather forthcoming about their preferences in bed and expect their partners to be the same. Their optimistic, fun-loving energy also makes them enthusiastic lovers who are down to do it anywhere, anytime, and any way.

Certainly those with Mars in Sagittarius are adventurous in bed, which gives them a playful, naughty streak. These are the lovers who will do it outside, in the bathroom, or upside down—you name it. They love a good game of cat and mouse, as long as it doesn't play out for *too* long. As with any fire sign, they are a bit impatient and are ready to cut to the chase. Fuck now, talk about it later.

Sagittarius rules over the hips and thighs, which makes these erogenous zones for these lovers. Mars in Sagittarius loves big hips and big thighs and is sure to grab a handful. Because Sagittarius is connected to foreign lands and cultures, Mars in Sagittarius babes love a good accent and may prefer to hook up with people from other countries or differing cultural backgrounds, similar to those with Venus in this sign.

No matter what, though, those with Mars in Sagittarius like to keep things lighthearted. No matter how serious they may be about someone, they will never want anything too overdone or emotional. They would much rather make you laugh all the way to the bedroom.

Truth be told, this is maybe one of the most chill placements for Mars. Frankly, Sagittarius is not interested in fighting and is the least likely of all the Mars signs to get into a confrontation. Will they debate you over an issue? Oh yeah. But getting into an actual screaming match? Unlikely. They simply cannot be bothered with such things. They are more likely to ghost you and move on to something or someone more exciting. Because Sagittarius uses humor to cope (or deflect) and is able to keep everything in perspective, it's pretty rare to actually see an angry Sagittarius Mars, or truly any Sagittarius placement at all.

MARS IN CAPRICORN

In Capricorn, we find Mars in the sign of its exaltation. As a reminder, the sign of a planet's exaltation is characterized by that sign sharing many of the same motivations and characteristics as that planet. In this case, we see the powerful drive and ambition of Capricorn shine through the lens of Mars. Capricorns are forever armed with a plan to achieve their goals and possess the practical wherewithal to make shit happen, so when this sign is paired with the planet of action, it creates a formidable force of will. There is an inherent dominance that exists within a Capricorn Mars. These lovers are in charge and they know it, and this is exactly the energy they bring to the bedroom.

That's right, Mars in Capricorn lovers are the daddies of the zodiac. Just as with everything else, they wield a well-developed know-how and authority and aren't afraid to assert themselves in the bedroom. They may, in fact, thrive on a bit of control and be attracted to powerful partners who can meet them blow for blow—or, in this case, maybe stroke for stroke. You can count on whatever Mars in Capricorn does in bed to be done well and to the best of their abilities. Their sexual prowess is deep and powerful, and they much prefer a constant, consistent partner over lots of variety. Remember that security is of the utmost importance to these lovers, and they require a feeling of security to express the full breadth of their erotic nature.

Those with Mars in Capricorn are rather private. This sign prefers discretion and isn't one for grand public displays. While these lovers may hold your hand in public, the beast isn't truly unleashed until they get you behind closed doors. And thanks to Mars being exalted in this sign, there's lots and lots of vitality to express.

Whereas an Aries Mars explodes like a fiery volcano, a Mars in Capricorn's anger is full of ice. Even at their most furious, there is a levelheadedness to their anger. These lovers possess an insane amount of self-control and therefore keep a tight leash on their rage. However, that doesn't mean being on the receiving end of their anger is any fun. As hard as they can be on themselves, they're going to be even harder on you if they're pissed.

Trust that Mars in Capricorn is going to be direct AF, and, similar to what we see with Mars in Virgo, their observations are devastatingly correct. Taking personal responsibility for whatever it is you've done is the fastest way to deescalate the situation.

MARS IN AQUARIUS

The cool, calm, and collected nature of Aquarius extends itself to Mars, giving these lovers a rather detached approach to sex. They have a "take it or leave it" attitude that, depending upon someone's personality, can be either wildly attractive or downright infuriating.

To be honest, this is probably the least passionate position of Mars. Their approach to sex is rather laissez-faire and, in true Aquarian fashion, will get filtered through the lens of intellectualizing. As I've mentioned before, Aquarius tends to love the *idea* of sex more than the actual act. Because of this, they're the most turned on or intrigued when the other person isn't or when their partner isn't around. Detachment is hot to them, period. This is why things like cybersex and phone sex are a big thing for those with Mars in Aquarius. Some of them may even be into hidden affairs, as a lot of them have fantasies about getting caught.

The irony here is that Mars in Aquarius lovers view themselves as being rather open-minded! Their fantasies and ideals around sex may be a bit odd or go against the grain, which is why we see polyamory, group sex, and other forms of nonmonogamy play a big role under the Aquarian influence.

Keep in mind, however, that those with Mars in Aquarius wield a formidable will, which can actually make them quite dominant in bed. However, because of their cool, casual way of doing things, you might not even notice how dominant they are at times!

When you've pissed off an Aquarius Mars, you'll know it. These lovers are the champions of shutting down and shutting out. Though they're pretty slow to anger, once they've been pushed far enough, Mars in Aquarius turns into a brick wall, just as we've seen with Mars in Taurus and Sagittarius. They are likely to isolate and take a ton of space, probably for longer than you'd like. Remember that Aquarius *is* a fixed sign, and therefore Mars here possesses the hallmark stubbornness of this sign, and there will simply be no talking to them until they've had a chance to cool down. The silent treatment is the name of the game for these folks, and the more frustrated you get, the harder they'll double down, and probably enjoy it, too.

MARS IN PISCES

Even though Mars isn't technically debilitated in the sign of Pisces, the red planet does tend to struggle here. Mars wants to be assertive and aggressive, but Pisces is far too sensitive for all that. While one of Pisces's superpowers is empathy, that quality can be detrimental when it comes time for these folks to stand up for themselves or take action.

This same subtle approach is taken when it comes to sex. While Mars in Pisces lovers are open to all forms of sexual expression, they definitely need a partner who is going to make the first move. Once that happens, they are true chameleon lovers. Mars in Pisces very much wants to please and will shape-shift into whatever form they need to become their partner's fantasy in real life. Because of this, their true sexual nature, as well as their real preferences in bed, can be difficult to pin down, though the fluid nature of their sexuality can be quite cool when honored in all its different forms.

Similar to what we see with Mars in Cancer, Pisces Mars lovers are die-hard romantics and are very soft, sweet, tender lovers. They can be freaky with the best of 'em, but at the end of the day they are looking to blur the lines between themselves and their partner and unite on a soul level. Trust that they want to snuggle and share plenty of sweet kisses. As Pisces rules over the feet, this is where we see the notorious foot fetish play out in real life.

Similar to Mars in Libra, a pissed-off Mars in Pisces will say something passive-aggressive. As much as these lovers may seem to go with the flow, they can stir up all kinds of trouble through an indirect manner. They aren't above playing games when they're pissed off, either, which can make them a bit manipulative where they are normally pretty peaceful, forgiving creatures. However, even the most passive of the bunch gets mad sometimes, and that aggression has to come out somehow. They can be a bit moody due to getting their feelings hurt easily, and the best way to neutralize their moods is definitely through some kind of creative outlet.

Keep in mind that because Mars in Pisces lovers have probably offered up an almost unending amount of compassion and understanding before finally getting angry enough to do something about it, extending that same understanding to them in return is the best way to get them to settle down.

A NOTE ON THE HOUSES

The house that Mars sits in within the chart first denotes an area of our lives where we see constant action. For example, a person with their Mars in the fourth house may have a busy family life and/or be someone who moves a lot or is constantly doing home improvement projects. Someone with their Mars in the fifth house may have lots of creative projects going on. Put simply, our Mars house is the area of our lives where we expend a lot of energy.

The second component of Mars in a house can indicate where we experience a lot of conflict. For example, someone with their Mars in the seventh house may have partnerships colored by a lot of arguments or struggle. However, the healthiest manifestation of conflict is what we fight *for*, not against.

Another way Mars might show up in the seventh house is fighting to keep the close relationships we value or fiercely protecting our partners in some way. In the course of a lifetime, it can be all these things.

Through a sexual lens, the house Mars sits in can show how and where and sometimes with whom our sexual energy shows up the most. Mars in the first house is someone who readily embodies their sexual prowess and is likely quite confident about it, whereas someone with Mars buried in the twelfth house may struggle to assert themselves or even be in touch with their sexual nature.

In the natal chart, the sixth house is the house of joy for Mars. Interestingly, ancient astrologers dubbed this house "Bad Fortune." When we consider that Mars is one of the two malefics in astrology, maybe this title makes more sense. However, it is a far cry from the associations of this house, which include our everyday, mundane lives, our routines, our job, and—where the Martian associations are the most obvious—our physical health. The Lesser Malefic is *busy* and therefore thrives within the bounds of the sixth house, which has us moving about, attending to all the demands of our daily lives. However, as Mars rejoices in moving the physical body, it also makes sense that Mars loves to be here.

The sixth house is yet another area where we see people attracted to the body. Because lovers with Mars here are prone to being health-conscious and are likely to take care of their body, this is an area where we see lots of athletes who, you guessed it, are hot.

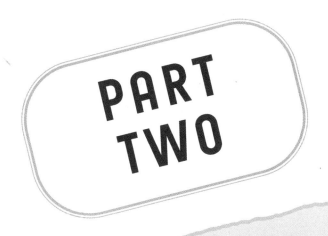

PART TWO

THE SOCIAL PLANETS

In astrology, the two social planets act as a bridge between the personal planets and the outer ones. This category—comprising only Jupiter and Saturn—is where we begin to look at transits on a longer scale and therefore begin to see larger groups of people with the same natal placements, the implications of which are interesting to consider through the lens of sextrology. There exists an innate similarity in the erotic nature of these groups of people who were born close together, even if only on a subtle level. This makes sense considering these people grew up together within the bounds of the same cultural trends, education, and messages around sex. The social planets enable us to zoom out a bit and see a bigger picture playing out within the sociocultural landscape at any given time.

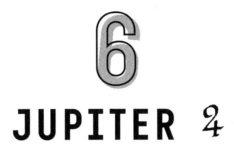

JUPITER ♃

DOMICILE: Sagittarius and Pisces

EXALTATION: Cancer

DETRIMENT: Gemini and Virgo

FALL: Capricorn

As we disembark from Mars's domain and enter into the riches of Jupiter's castle, we leave behind the personal planets and enter the territory of the social planets: Jupiter and Saturn. Jupiter is the first time we see people grouped together in larger ways. The Greater Benefic spends about a year transiting a sign, and thus everyone born within the same twelve-month period will have the same Jupiter placement in their charts. This is where we begin to see larger numbers of people all grouped into the same sign, creating a similarity across any given cohort, regardless of their personal placements. What kinds of implications does this have when thinking about love and sex?

In sextrology, the abundance of Jupiter translates into the ways we seek new, expansive experiences in our sex lives. It points to the adventurous part of ourselves that seeks to learn more through gaining more experiences with more people. Jupiter always wants more, more, more.

JUPITER IN ARIES

In Aries, the first sign of the zodiac, Jupiter's abundance and expansion come through the avenue of passion—specifically, through embodying our passion.

The trick to understanding Jupiter is that when we embrace and act out the characteristics of the sign it falls in within our charts, we get rewarded. In the case of Jupiter in Aries, those rewards are dished out when these lovers heed their passionate side, take action, embrace their individuality, and get clear about their wants, needs, and desires. Expansion comes through vitality, the hunt, being up-front about who and what they want, and being bold about it. Remember that Aries is an incredibly physical sign, and abundance lies within this physicality as well. Honoring this primal part of themselves and expressing their passions through the flesh will unlock many riches.

Aries lovers are clear and uncompromising about their desires and are fueled by the fires of desire that burn within. For these people, following that spark is key, as is cultivating some self-love and figuring out how to be unapologetic about who they are and what they want. This same philosophy shows up when thinking about expanding their erotic experiences: Be bold, direct, and forward about who and what you want. Go big or go home.

JUPITER IN TAURUS

Whenever the planet of abundance rests its laurels in Taurus, good fortune comes through slowing down. Taurus is the sign that wants to douse itself in sensual experiences: relishing every bite, luxuriating in a hot bath or shower, savoring the smell of fresh laundry. Taurus wants to stop and smell the roses, literally and figuratively.

For these lovers, abundance comes through doing the same. Be careful, though, as Jupiter can lend itself to overindulgence, gluttony, and prioritizing pleasure over everything else! There is such a thing as too much of a good thing. Remember that Taurus is also the master of boundaries.

Certainly expansiveness comes for those with Jupiter in Taurus through embracing their sensual side, period. Patience and taking their time both in and out of the bedroom will open up their world. But, yes, slow sex that is deeply sensual is key. Stamina is too. Taurus is a sign that can and will go all night long, and there's something about indulging in the flesh for as long as they want that will truly fill their cup.

JUPITER IN GEMINI

Jupiter is considered to be in detriment in Gemini, the first of the Mercury-ruled signs. Jupiter focuses on the big picture in life, desiring a heaven-high vantage point in order to be able to maintain the correct perspective on things. Gemini, on the other hand, focuses on the details, seeking to acquire as much information as possible before being able to make a decision. Also—no offense, Gemini—but the astral twins tend to struggle with committing to and following through on things. Gemini's insatiable curiosity often leaves them feeling interested in everything and therefore nothing, and for Jupiter this simply won't do.

Regardless, Jupiter brings expansion through curiosity: Gemini's mind is voracious, and those with their natal Jupiter here are the same. Gemini knows that variety is the spice of life, and they don't see any need to box themselves into any one thing. With Gemini it's "yes, and," not "either/or."

This same philosophy extends to sex and romance. Embracing their desire for variety, and many different types of lovers, experiences, and kinds of relationships, is important for Jupiter in Gemini. Fluidity is a great keyword, too. Because of Gemini's ability to see things from all sides and to adapt accordingly, remaining open and curious about love, sex, relationship types, and even their own sexuality is key for these lovers. Maintaining a bit of that awe and wonder and allowing themselves to explore and experience any type of connection will open the gates of abundance.

JUPITER IN CANCER

Cardinal water sign Cancer has been gifted the title of exaltation where Jupiter is concerned. As with all exalted planets, there are lots of similarities between the characteristics of Cancer and those of Jupiter, which creates a certain amount of ease and power here.

Those with their Jupiter in Cancer are kind, loving, and nurturing souls. They tend to be quite generous and possess a strong spiritual side that comes paired with an equally strong intuition. Because Jupiter is all about growth, the TLC of Cancer lends itself well to the goals of the Greater Benefic. All things grow with a little love and attention, and nobody knows that better than a person with their Jupiter here.

Through the lens of sextrology, abundance and expansion come through fostering the safety and security that can only come through emotional intimacy that has been cultivated over time. This doesn't mean these lovers are incapable of casual sex, but true abundance comes where the emotional piece matches the physical.

Generosity is a key component here as well. More than any other position of Jupiter, Cancer Jupiter lovers experience abundance through giving. The more they give, the more they receive, and this dynamic extends to sex! Something about being givers in the bedroom unlocks their ability to receive as well. Because of their keen intuition, these lovers are naturally in tune with their partners, knowing exactly what they like and being ready and willing to deliver. Through this exchange, they will begin to receive generously from others, too.

JUPITER IN LEO

In Leo, Jupiter leaves behind its position of exaltation in Cancer and takes on a much different face. Those with this Jupiter placement are creative and magnetic and make fabulous leaders. The name of the game is self-expression, through which Leo thrives in channeling their creativity and dramatic flair. The abundance of Jupiter is unlocked through Leo's passions and warmhearted nature, especially when these lovers are generous, bold, and acting from a place of authenticity.

When it comes to sextrology, I again want to emphasize that Leo is the sign associated with sex. Therefore, for people with Jupiter in Leo, embodying their natural prowess and playfulness is the avenue to expansion and growth. More so than for any other sign, except for maybe Aries, being themselves allows Leo lovers to shine. There is also something essential that lies in allowing themselves to shine in all the things that set them apart. Their uniqueness is their superpower, and there's something about bringing that energy into the bedroom that will be greatly fulfilling. Also, don't forget to be bold about it!

JUPITER IN VIRGO

In Virgo, the second of the Mercury-ruled signs, Jupiter is also in detriment. As we saw with Jupiter in Gemini, Jupiter thrives on a big-picture perspective, and thanks to its Mercurial nature, Virgo is often swept up in the minutiae of it all. This is a sign that thrives on the details: They want it, they need it, and they're going to get it. Unlike Gemini, however, Virgo definitely has the follow-through. These individuals are pragmatic, ambitious, organized, and service-oriented.

The expansive nature of Jupiter manifests for these lovers through the aforementioned qualities as well as the avenue of health. Especially where sextrology is concerned, prioritizing healthy sex practices is key for Jupiter in Virgo. Taking the time to engage in whatever routines they need around sex will cultivate a feeling of joy and abundance for these lovers. Maybe that doesn't sound very exciting, but it's true, and taking the time to manicure yourself and nurture your body will be deeply fulfilling, so much so that it may surprise you. And, yes, that means using whatever means of protection you prefer during sex.

Beyond this, sexual sovereignty comes forward. Because Virgo placements often struggle with their own sexuality and how their beliefs around sex differ from those around them, finding a way to be rooted in themselves when it comes to sex is highly, highly effective. Embracing sexual sovereignty means owning your erotic nature, no matter what it looks like or whether or not you're sleeping with someone. Try it out.

JUPITER IN LIBRA

In the sign of the scales, Jupiter shows its face through balance, fairness, and equality in all things. As with any Libra placement, Jupiter in Libra places an emphasis on relationships, and in fact partnership may be the avenue through which abundance and expansion are achieved. However, the emphasis here is on treating others fairly and using the Libra grace and charm within their relationships. Equality, kindness, and fairmindedness are the focus. The age-old adage "Treat others as you want to be treated" was coined for this placement.

Again we see Jupiter through the Venusian lens in Libra, so pleasure, beauty, the arts, and creativity are also favored. Embracing and cultivating all Venusian faculties while also maintaining a strong sense of balance and fairness is the key to unlocking the good fortune of Jupiter here.

When thinking about Jupiter in Libra in relation to sex, it truly is relationships that will help to unlock and expand your sexual nature. Learning the art of giving and receiving both in and out of the bedroom is a must. Everything must be mutual, including pleasure.

JUPITER IN SCORPIO

Intensity, passion, and desire are the name of the game when Jupiter is in Scorpio. More than for any other Jupiter placement, these lovers get rewarded when they put their all into something. Remember that Scorpio doesn't do anything by halves. They operate in extremes, so you're either all in or all out. And in this case, you better be all in.

Following the paths that are lit by the flames of passion is the only way for Jupiter in Scorpio. These may be the deeper and/or darker things in life, such as psychology, anything taboo or mysterious, and the occult. Uncovering mysteries and secrets is Scorpio's specialty, after all.

Beyond that, figuring out how to turn up your personal magnetism in order to attract whatever and whoever you desire can bring plenty of choices and opportunities.

This same idea extends to sex as well. Scorpio rules over the genitals and is highly sexual by nature. Embracing the passionate, borderline obsessive, and physical side of yourself is truly what will bring expansion. Maybe that feels a little too on the nose, but it's true. Scorpio's sexual appetite knows no bounds, so honor the voraciousness within.

JUPITER IN SAGITTARIUS

Jupiter finds itself at home within the bounds of the cosmic archer, whose very lifeblood is learning through experience. Sagittarius possess an incredible zest for life, seeking to expand their literal and figurative horizons through as many different kinds of experiences as they can pack into one lifetime. When it comes to sextrology, Jupiter in Sagittarius quite literally speaks to gaining more experience.

Now, if you have Jupiter in Sagittarius, this doesn't have to mean that you're destined to sleep with a bunch of people—though it can, if you want. It's more about welcoming in the spirit of adventure where sex is concerned and being open to trying new things. Remember that Sagittarius thrives on fun and humor. Allowing those elements to come into play both in and out of the bedroom will unlock a whole new world for you and will help to cultivate ease and a sense of abundance in your love life.

JUPITER IN CAPRICORN

Despite the wisdom that is often assigned to Capricorn (something that is often ascribed to the Greater Benefic itself), Jupiter is considered to be in its fall in this sign. This is simply due to the fact that Jupiter rules over all things spiritual and otherworldly; the intangible is truly Jupiter's bread and butter. Capricorn, on the other hand, is an earth sign whose very existence is rooted deep in the tangible. Where Jupiter asks for a leap of faith, Capricorn would rather place their bet on a well-formed plan.

Now, the curiosity of a seemingly ill-placed Jupiter is that we still reap the abundance promised by this planet through embodying the qualities of the sign it falls in, in this case the ideals of Capricorn. These lovers attract the most good fortune when they are organized, pragmatic, ethical, and mature. As always, we're seeking to really live in our integrity here, and while doing that is a good idea for everyone, it's especially true for these babes. Streamlining things and acting from a place of authority is also a good idea.

Cultivating abundance around your eroticism comes through embracing the authority within, too—which means being in charge in the bedroom!

Capricorn is dominant, period, and even for those who may be a bit shy or timid when it comes to sex, Jupiter wants them to give it a shot. Don't forget to stay true to your values, though! Even in the more overt aspects of dominance, it's still important to have good aftercare.

JUPITER IN AQUARIUS

In Aquarius, Jupiter takes on an eccentric nature. In a way, Jupiter is placed quite well in this sign, as both the planet and the water bearer are all about freedom. Especially through the Aquarian lens, the key for this Jupiter placement is tolerance and being able not only to take their own personal space but also to give it to others. Any of the liberties these people want or need for themselves must also be given freely to everyone else.

Embracing the authentic self plays a central role with Jupiter in Aquarius, similar to Jupiter in Aries and Leo. Everything that makes these lovers unique, different, and innovative gets amped up under Jupiter's watch, and, more importantly, embodying those traits and ideals unlocks a great deal of ease and good fortune.

This same idea leads to growth and expansion in relationships, too. Aquarius often harbors some pretty different ideas about love, sex, and romance, and living a life in alignment with those values will unlock the abundance they seek. If you want to try out polyamory, do it. If you don't believe in the institution of marriage, don't get married. If you want to move to a commune and own goats and have your children raised by a community, buy a plot of land. There's no idea or dream that is too weird here. Let your freak flag fly.

JUPITER IN PISCES

The final sign of the zodiac is where we find Jupiter in its second home. As I've noted in a few other places in this book, Pisces is the most spiritual of all the signs. They are all about empathy, compassion, and service and possess a powerful faith in the Divine and the goodness of all people. There is a huge focus on creativity, generosity, and an idealistic universal vision for humanity. Whenever these lovers act from a place of unconditional love and understanding, their lives open up in new and beautiful ways.

With Jupiter in Pisces, sexual expansion and abundance come from embracing the fluidity of their sexual expression. Pisces lovers in particular are full of fantasy and romance and prefer to mold themselves around whatever it is their partner likes in the bedroom. Because of this, their erotic nature can take on innumerable forms. Honoring the constant metamorphosis of their sexuality to bend and change and shapeshift into whatever form it wants to take will open the door to abundance, ecstasy, and fulfillment.

A NOTE ON THE HOUSES

Understanding the influence of Jupiter in the twelve houses deviates from the way we think about having other planets in a particular house. Because Jupiter is the planet of abundance and ease, the house it lives in points to the area of our lives where we experience such ease. It may be an area where we are viewed as being particularly lucky, and indeed we might be.

For example, someone who has their Jupiter in the tenth house is viewed favorably by people in positions of authority. They are generally well-liked and held in high esteem by their bosses, managers, and the community at large. This is also someone who has an unusually large number of good opportunities fall into their lap by way of their career. It may seem like they just happen to be in the right place at the right time, somehow always meeting the right people who have the right connections and want to hire them for the job. In that same vein, if they manage to score an interview somewhere, 99.9 percent of the time they snag the gig.

As another example, someone with their Jupiter in the seventh house of serious romantic relationships is never short of potential lovers. They attract people with ease, seeming to do almost nothing and somehow being forever wildly popular with the people they prefer to date. They may seem to always be in a serious relationship, whereas others may struggle to attract even one mate.

Now, it's also important to keep in mind that others may not necessarily view us as being deserving of such abundance, and to a certain extent maybe that's true. However, as we all have Jupiter influencing our lives somehow, we must be careful when pointing the finger, as we wind up with three other fingers pointing right back at us!

The planet of abundance finds its joy in the eleventh house, dubbed "Good Spirit" by the ancients. Again, as Jupiter is the second of the two benefics in astrology, and the greater one at that, the natural association of this planet with "good" makes sense. As the eleventh is the house of community and also of hopes, dreams, and the future, Jupiter loves to bring its optimism and larger-than-life nature to this area of our lives.

Similar to Jupiter in the tenth house, and perhaps even more so, those with Jupiter in the eleventh house are hugely popular. They probably have a huge network of people they know and are generally adored by their community. Plus, they love to connect with people and often benefit from their many networks in some way. These lovers are altruistic and focused on the greater good, able to see optimistic views of the future and bring their own natural talents to their various social groups.

7

SATURN ♄

DOMICILE: Capricorn and Aquarius

EXALTATION: Libra

DETRIMENT: Cancer and Leo

FALL: Aries

Saturn, the Greater Malefic, spends even longer in a sign than Jupiter does, around two and half years. Similar to Jupiter placements, this creates the same Saturn placement for those born within two-ish years of one another, creating an even larger group than the former. As the final of the seven traditional planets and the second of the two social planets, Saturn truly enacts its main quality of boundaries, acting as a cosmic threshold before we move on to the generational planets, Uranus, Neptune, and Pluto.

In sextrology, this heavy hitter manifests as the foundation of our erotic nature, where we seek to build stability and sustainability around sexuality, as well as the limitations we experience. Saturn is ultimately the way we doubt ourselves, and therefore it points to the maturation we need to experience to overcome these insecurities. Saturn teaches us that sex gets better with time.

SATURN IN ARIES

We kick off the journey of Saturn through the signs with Aries, where it's in its fall. Because Saturn is concerned more with society at large, it makes sense that since Aries is the sign of the self, there are plenty of differing motivations where Aries is concerned that make it difficult for Saturn to express itself here the way it desires. In this case, we see limitations and fears around expressing and asserting oneself. These lovers may struggle to take action and/or face conflict. There is a certain stifling around their natural aggression, anger, and competitive side. Certainly where sextrology is concerned, the Saturn in Aries group has issues around self-pleasure and anything that might be viewed as selfish vis-à-vis their wants and needs in the bedroom and with their sexual expression in general, making the karma of Saturn the most overtly related to sex in this sign.

SATURN IN TAURUS

Through the lens of Taurus, Saturnian themes manifest through resources and pleasure. We can see fears rooted in attaining and maintaining material stability and security, as well as through any kind of indulgence or the need to move slowly. Certainly, the slow-moving nature of both Taurus and Saturn is reinforced and makes any effort feel grueling and like trying to run through mud. However, because both Taurus and Saturn inherently point to stability, it's possible that these lovers are actually quite secure as far as money is concerned. The journey for these folks may be more about them breaking through any fear around scarcity and lack rather than them actually experiencing it. There's certainly a call to learn how to enjoy the rewards of working hard rather than feeling guilty about it, which is one way we see the idea of limitations around pleasure come through.

Without being able to access any type of pleasure or enjoyment, life becomes a series of burdens for Saturn in Taurus. The struggle around self-indulgence can lead to binging and purging cycles, going from moments of gluttony to periods of austerity. Ideally, over time these lovers learn to find the middle ground, cultivating a more sustainable practice around pleasure as they grow older.

This same idea extends to sex. For Saturn in Taurus, there are plenty of lessons around control, power, and excess when it comes to matters of the flesh, which are probably more self-imposed than anything. Journeying toward true sustainability happens through redefining their relationship to sensuality, pleasure, and abundance. There also may be some destigmatizing that needs to happen from whatever values they were taught in adolescence.

SATURN IN GEMINI

In curious Gemini, heavy-hitting Saturn turns its sights on communication, learning, sharing, and connection. As the first mutable sign in the zodiac, Gemini brings a welcome flexibility to the normally rigid and unbending will of the Greater Malefic. This brings a certain ease to this placement that those with Saturn in other signs may not experience—but, as our experiences are all subjective, that doesn't mean these lovers find their journey with Saturn any less trying.

Ultimately, those with Saturn in Gemini struggle with limitations around expressing themselves, especially when it comes to expressing their curious, lighthearted, or enthusiastic side. They may feel bothered by those who talk too much or seem to lead vapid, superficial lives, but this is likely a projection of their own fears or limitations. Through the lens of Gemini, Saturn manifests as being guarded in speech and/or the written word, which forces these individuals to work extra hard in all things related to communication. They may also be extra sensitive to criticism, as Saturn instills them with a sharp inner critic that demands nothing less than perfection.

In sextrology, these lovers must work hard to be able to communicate their desires and perspectives around sex and all things erotic. For those with Saturn in Gemini, learning to ask for what they want in a clear and effective way takes practice and may feel especially difficult, as their desires and needs change constantly, in true Gemini fashion. Learning to lean into their versatility and fluidity is key here, as is learning to embrace other perspectives and approaches to love and sex. There may be some preconceived notions or stigmas around sex that need to get dismantled before true expression can come forward.

SATURN IN CANCER

In sensitive Cancer, the opposite sign of Capricorn, Saturn is in its first sign of detriment. Because Saturn demands personal responsibility and hard work on our part and Cancer is about nurturing and giving and receiving support from family and close loved ones, the desires of this pairing are fundamentally at odds. This isn't to say that Cancers aren't hard workers. On the contrary, they are one of the four cardinal signs, and in that sense they make great leaders, organizers, and initiators. But when we think about the traditional societal norms of Saturn, especially through the lens of Capricorn, Cancer is often the manifestation of emotional labor and/or the work that is done by homemakers—work that isn't exactly valued the way it ought to be (which says more about society than stay-at-home parents).

Regardless, those with this position of Saturn struggle to get their emotional needs met. They may feel abandoned or left to their own devices when what they truly need is support and understanding from others. Keep in mind that this feeling of being left out in the cold may be self-imposed, however, as the hallmark of Saturn in Cancer is to fortify their shell of armor to protect their vulnerable side. Because Cancer has a tendency to dwell on past hurts, they may end up in a vicious cycle of a self-fulfilling prophecy where they shut people out before they can get hurt instead of leaving the door open to let others help. They may end up holding things in, thinking they can depend only on themselves, and end up harboring resentment that need not exist in the first place. Certainly the call here is to learn how to let other people in.

As with all Cancer placements, Saturn in Cancer's sexual journey pertains to emotional intimacy and its tie to sex. Intimacy is an actual need for these lovers, but first they've got to learn how to risk making themselves vulnerable in this way before they can actually have the deep connections they seek. Because Cancer rules over the family of origin, there are likely messages they received about sex growing up that need to be dismantled as well.

SATURN IN LEO

In bold-as-hell Leo, Saturn is in the second sign of its detriment, as Leo is the opposite sign of Aquarius, the other sign that Saturn rules. Just as we experience Saturn at home in back-to-back signs, so do we experience Saturn in detriment back-to-back. Similar to what we just saw with Saturn in

Cancer, Saturn in Leo is a placement where we see yet another diametrically opposed set of desires between heavy-hitting Saturn and charismatic Leo. In this case, the juxtaposition exists between the humanitarian, collective focus of Aquarius and the individual-focused nature of Leo.

Those with Saturn in Leo are forced to reckon with their need for attention, validation, and approval. In fact, for whatever reason, their default may be to not call attention to themselves, completely denying their true need to show off their talents and unique characteristics. Certainly there is also a journey for them around joy, playfulness, creativity, and empowering the inner child. There also may be issues around authority and feeling controlled by others, which Leo downright hates.

At some point these lovers are going to have to grapple with their desire for self-expression and the insecurities that keep them from feeling confident enough to show up authentically. The limitations of Saturn do make it hard for them to just be themselves, but with some hard work and commitment, they can overcome this.

On the sextrology front, we again see the question of sex as being quite literal with Saturn in Leo. These babes have a fear of expressing their sexuality as boldly and freely as they'd truly like. Embodying their erotic nature to the fullest is the call here, but there are likely some beliefs around worthiness, confidence, and maybe just sex in general that have to get dismantled first. Confronting their limitations around deserving pleasure is a big deal for those with this placement.

SATURN IN VIRGO

With Saturn in hyper-responsible Virgo, we see a journey around work and all the responsibilities and demands of daily life. As Virgo is the second of the four mutable signs, we again see the potential here for greater fluidity than with other Saturn positions, though it's important to keep in mind that Virgo struggles greatly with control and perfectionism, which can be amplified under Saturn's influence.

The main manifestation of Saturn in Virgo is someone who takes on way more responsibility than they should. Because Virgo is the sign of service, they are always looking to help, and this often ends up with them saying yes when they need to say no. Especially because Saturn is about responsibility and hard work, burnout from the burden of too many responsibilities is a real possibility here. Criticism, especially of the self, can turn especially sharp and insidious as well, as it is hard for these individuals to let something go if it doesn't feel exactly perfect.

Virgo is notorious for having high standards, and with the limitations of Saturn, those standards can quite literally become impossible to reach. At some point in their lives, these lovers are going to have to grapple with what is actually achievable and realistic. What are we truly capable of? What are *they* truly capable of? And where the heck do they need better boundaries?

Through the lens of sextrology, Saturn in Virgo is about creating routines and structure around sexual health and wellness. This may not be something that was instilled in these individuals growing up, so they must take on the responsibility of prioritizing it for themselves. Because Virgo is often quite nervous and insecure when it comes to sex, there may also be some dismantling around their sexual performance that needs to happen as well. Ultimately, Saturn in Virgo is about finding joy in routines and daily life and, by extension, finding joy and fulfillment in sex, too.

SATURN IN LIBRA

Saturn finds the space of its exaltation in justice-oriented Libra. Because Saturn is all about rules and regulations, it makes sense that the Greater Malefic thrives in the sign that is all about what's fair and right, especially through a higher lens that transcends subjectivity, instead wishing to establish a set of norms that apply to all people, regardless of status, power, money, creed, etc. Certainly those with Saturn in Libra have a well-developed sense of what's fair, what's right, and what justice and equality truly mean.

As with all Libra placements, Saturn in Libra puts relationships front and center. These lovers take relationships very seriously and are ready to commit. However, their sense of responsibility to others can be so strong that they have a hard time letting go of bad connections and/or welcoming in new ones. Loneliness is also a big theme here, as these babes are forced to grapple with the "self versus other" push-pull dynamics of relationships that may leave them desiring independence only to regret it later.

For those with Saturn in Libra, sexual maturity comes through dismantling what they believe makes a relationship fair and balanced. At some point, with age and experience, they will have to grapple with their own definition of equality, of give-and-take, of a healthy and balanced relationship. Boundaries in love are especially important here, and through this reconstruction they are able to redefine their idea of commitment, too. This same philosophy extends to the bedroom, with these individuals needing to find partnerships with an equal amount of give-and-take and where they are not always the one who gives, gives, gives. Keep in mind that there may be some work that needs to be done around learning how to receive without feeling guilty or weird about it.

SATURN IN SCORPIO

In heavily guarded Scorpio, Saturn amplifies the mistrust and fear of this sign around emotional vulnerability. These lovers have a hard time dealing with their deeper, more intense emotions. Oftentimes these feelings, such as jealousy, are viewed as irrational or negative, and there is a desire to limit or stifle them. However, doing so really only stifles the full spectrum of human emotions, self-expression, and experience. Besides, trying to ignore a feeling or stuff it down doesn't actually eradicate it. All it does is make those unprocessed feelings come out sideways later on.

In fact, lovers with Saturn in Scorpio actually have a strong desire for deep emotional intimacy, but they can struggle to admit that both to others and to themselves. Their Saturnian journey, therefore, involves learning how to fully open themselves up to others in order to experience the depth that Scorpio craves. Learning how to embrace the transformative power of change is also a necessity and is something that goes hand in hand with finding true intimacy. Without being open to being changed through connecting deeply with another, satisfaction will be something that evades them forever.

It should be no surprise, then, that for Saturn in Scorpio, maturity comes through intimacy, period. There is a need to confront the resistance and fear they have around sex, intimacy, and deep emotional connections. Those with Saturn in Scorpio require a dismantling around the taboo nature of sex that was instilled in them growing up—whatever that means—and instead need to learn to embrace the passion, the desire, the ardor in all its beauty. Sex isn't something to be ashamed of but rather embraced, if we hope to have any kind of healthy, truly fulfilling experience with it. There is likely some sexual shame at the root of it all that these lovers will be forced to confront and evolve away from. For Saturn in Scorpio, embracing the vulnerability that inherently exists around sex can actually lead to unlocking a powerful eroticism and animal magnetism that is yearning to come to the surface and breathe.

SATURN IN SAGITTARIUS

In exuberant Sagittarius, Saturn brings forward questions around freedom, exploration, religion, and beliefs. Thanks to Sagittarius being a mutable sign, we don't see the same rigidity we're used to with Saturn in a fixed sign or in Capricorn. Instead, Saturn becomes flexible and malleable here and allows for more breathing room where systems and structures are concerned. That said, the question of rigidity is an important one with this placement.

In a twist of irony, those with Saturn in Sagittarius can be quite stuck in their ways when it comes to their perspectives! These lovers prefer to live by their own rules and can therefore be quite skeptical when presented with alternative beliefs. This position of Saturn tends to manifest one of two ways: either by subscribing to a rigid belief system (such as a religion) or by rejecting organized systems of belief altogether. At one point or another—perhaps during the infamous Saturn return—their faith is going to be tested and they will end up questioning what they've believed in so ardently. At the end of the day, Sagittarius has a need to understand the "why" behind things, and until these individuals can find an answer that satisfies them, they may struggle to feel balanced and grounded.

For those with Saturn in Sagittarius, sexual maturity comes through actually embodying the beliefs they so furiously subscribe to when it comes to love and relationships. More so than for any other position of Saturn, their journey is quite literally about learning through experience. Saturn in Sagittarius lovers need time to explore their philosophy around all things erotic in order to truly develop and understand what they believe in and hold to be true. The wisdom that is gained through experience and can only come with age plays out here in a way we don't really see anywhere else. These folks will likely end up taking on a completely new perspective when it comes to sex at some point in their lives. Learning to embrace a little more optimism and spontaneity can help them to open their minds.

SATURN IN CAPRICORN

The first of Saturn's home signs is Capricorn, the astral sea goat. This cardinal earth sign thrives on all things Saturnian, including rules, structure, wisdom, and knowing the value of working toward something over the long term. Capricorn knows how to commit and appreciates the weight and value of responsibility. They know what it means to show up time and again, acting as a reliable mountain of stability. There is something inherently traditional about Capricorn that we don't see with any other sign.

When approaching this placement of Saturn in sextrology, we end up looking to the family of origin and what was modeled for us growing up. What kind of relationship did your parents have? What kind of values were ingrained in you through them? What were the views around sex and love that were inevitably modeled for and imparted to you? For this group of Saturnians, grappling with these questions is inevitable. Eventually we all have to confront where we came from and what was taught to us, and eventually these individuals will have to decide if they want to perpetuate those traditions and values around relationships or not.

It's likely that, at least in the beginning, these people will find themselves experiencing and embodying, whether wittingly or unwittingly, the same patterns and dynamics of their parents. For Saturn in Capricorn, maturity comes through confronting and likely dismantling these "rules" and being able to discern what actually works for *them*, no matter what their family has to say about it.

I would like to underline the fact that Capricorn is more about breaking free from the foundational things that were modeled within the family and not necessarily within society, as we will see in Aquarius, though the two may look similar.

SATURN IN AQUARIUS

Just as the signs of Saturn's detriment are back-to-back, the signs of Saturn in domicile follow each other as well. Thus, we find Saturn moving straight into its second home in airy Aquarius. Both Capricorn and Aquarius are highly concerned with rules and structure, but where Capricorn seeks to implement rules, Aquarius seeks to dismantle them. Thus, through the lens of sextrology, we apply the journey of Saturn in Aquarius toward breaking down preconceived and indoctrinated notions around society's definition of what is normal, acceptable, and conventional where sex and love are concerned.

By now we've established that the inherent nature of Aquarius is subversive, seeking to try on everything new and cutting-edge in order to find new solutions that are more equal, fair, and accessible. For those with this position of Saturn, the limitations—and the maturity—come through embracing more equitable dynamics in their romantic and sexual connections. For example, perhaps they wind up with a partner who wants to open the relationship, or perhaps they're queer, or maybe the relationship is more asexual. The possibilities are endless, but there is something about embracing the unconventional and experimental that actually leads to growth and more sustainable foundations in relationships for those with Saturn in Aquarius. There is also a certain detachment that Aquarius asks for that can be helpful for the Saturn person. Being able to look at something through a purely objective, logical lens will be helpful here.

SATURN IN PISCES

At the end of the zodiac, Saturn departs from its back-to-back home placements and finds itself in Pisces, where it can essentially just chill. Saturn in Pisces is a bit of an enigma, though, as it seeks to bring form and structure to the formless waters of the cosmic fishes. The very nature of Pisces is formless, boundless, and ethereal. It is the sign that exists the most in the spirit world, the dreamscape, and pretty much anything that transcends the physical plane. In that sense, Pisces is fundamentally different from Saturn, which seeks to ground us deep into the earth.

In sextrology, Saturn is about being able to ground all the fantasies of Pisces into reality. As the romantics and dreamers of the zodiac, Pisces lovers have plenty of fantasies, sexually and otherwise, when it comes to their love lives. For those with Saturn in Pisces, maturity comes through being able to embrace these fantasies, no matter how taboo or kinky (or not), and turn them into something tangible. There is likely also a journey around figuring out what is actually realistic where their fantasies and expectations are concerned. Role-playing in the bedroom? Sure. Finding themselves a seven-foot-tall, magical, real-life elf? Probably not.

Beyond this, we also have to confront the giving, sacrificial nature of Pisces here. Any Pisces placement will default to their desire to give, and while it's perfectly fine to be a giver in the bedroom, that doesn't have to mean sex turns into a sacrificial act. With Saturn in Pisces, there may also be some anxiety around needing to be able to pleasure their partners, again in that same vein of service. While it's beautiful to care about your partner's pleasure, there is a line to be drawn and lessons to learn around being able to receive. Boundaries are especially important for those with this Saturn placement.

A NOTE ON THE HOUSES

A deeper understanding of Saturn's role in your chart comes through looking at the house it sits in, too. The themes and areas of life ruled by that house further color the lifelong karmic journey of Saturn and where we will have to grapple with its lessons time and again. The area of our lives indicated by Saturn's house placement denotes where we experience the obstacles and limitations we are constantly faced with, and in that sense, that area may feel especially difficult. Wherever Saturn shows up, we have to work extra hard and take on more responsibility. In astrology, the Greater Malefic rules over time, and many Saturnian lessons are literally a matter of time, meaning we can understand what Saturn is trying to teach us only with enough life experience and the wisdom that comes with age. Because of this, Saturn's lessons get easier as we get older. We cannot understand or appreciate the gifts and lessons of this planet until we are older. In that sense, we can also see the ways that experience in relationships grants us the wisdom Saturn seeks to impart as well.

The Greater Malefic is the only planet that finds its joy in the twelfth house. Hellenistic astrology calls this house "Bad Spirit," again in association with Saturn's "malevolent" nature. Note that Saturn marks the end of the planetary joys, as during the Hellenistic period only the seven traditional planets were known to exist!

As a rule, Saturn loves being behind the curtain of the twelfth house. Because this is a place of obscurity that exists just underneath the surface of our conscious awareness, Saturn can operate uninterrupted and tend to its many, unrelenting tasks free of interruption or distraction. The twelfth house is a place of solitude, and Saturn, by nature, is cold and distant, preferring to operate on its own, in the peace and quiet that solitude brings, creating a natural affinity between it and the final house of the birth chart. In the twelfth house, Saturn has plenty of time and space to reflect deeply and tend to debts, endings, and past issues that need resolution.

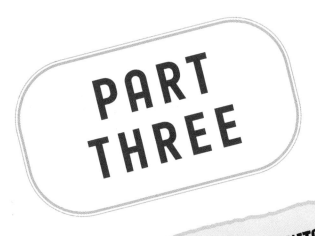

PART THREE

THE GENERATIONAL PLANETS

Finally we arrive at the threshold of the three outer, or generational, planets in astrology. Uranus, Neptune, and Pluto are the evolutionary trio that make up this category, and they're still pretty new to the scene in the long-standing practice of astrology. Only the hyper-modern branches of astrology include them, and sextrology happens to be one of them.

Even more so than with Jupiter and Saturn, the generational planets transit signs over a long period of time—sometimes for two decades or more—creating even larger groups of people with the same placements. The generational planets enable us to zoom out even further and see the collective shifts in attitude around sexuality in a real way.

On an individual level, unless an outer planet is strongly placed (say, conjunct the Ascendant, for example), its influence tends to be more subtle and is something we experience over the long run, as opposed to feeling the influence of the personal planets every single day. Again, the implications here are pretty interesting and are something I encourage you to reflect on as you make your way through this section. How have you seen or experienced the themes of your Uranus placement play out in your life thus far? Your Neptune? Pluto?

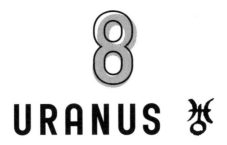

URANUS ⛢

MODERN-DAY RULER OF: Aquarius

HIGHER OCTAVE OF: Mercury

Our entrance into the electric field of Uranus marks yet another transition from the social planets into what are known as the generational planets in astrology: Uranus, Neptune, and Pluto. As the first of the generational planets, Uranus initiates us into an area of astrology that has a much longer-term influence than any of the other planets covered so far. Uranus, for example, spends a much longer time transiting a sign—around seven years. All together, Uranus's orbit around the Sun, and therefore through the zodiac, takes 84 years. Thanks to this longer stint in each sign, Uranus (and Neptune and Pluto) creates even larger "generations" than Saturn does.

The delineation often ascribed to the three generational planets is that we don't experience them in our day-to-day lives the same way we do the personal planets. This all depends on where these planets are placed in your chart, of course, but still, generally speaking that may be true. When we think about the roles of these planets in sextrology, they may in fact point to things we grapple with over a lifetime of exploring our sexuality rather than having their subjective experiences front and center. Again, it all depends on your personal chart.

In astrology, Uranus is the planet of radical change. It sweeps in at unexpected moments with shocking revelations that seem to undo everything in the blink of an eye. It is electrifying, exciting, and terrifying. As the modern-day ruler of Aquarius, Uranus is experimental, avant-garde, and outside the box. When thinking about this planet and its relationship to sex, we end up with a point in the chart that illuminates our desire for experimentation and exploration.

URANUS IN ARIES

I think the themes of Uranus and Aries blend together quite well. The call to embody your most radical, authentic self is something both Aries and Uranus are concerned with, and in this case radical change happens through your passions. With Uranus in Aries, being bold, courageous, and unapologetic about your wants, needs, and desires will set you free. Taking action toward anything that ignites the internal flames of passion acts as a catalyst to liberation.

What to Try in the Bedroom

- Embody your passion and desire for newness.
- Keep sex feeling fresh and fun.
- Honor your instincts and your raw, physical nature.
- Try playing the dominant role and be the one who does the pursuing.
- Live in the moment.
- Emphasize self-pleasure.
- Own your actual wants and needs, and be bold and courageous about voicing them.

URANUS IN TAURUS

The combination of Uranus and Taurus in the birth chart is a bit of an oxymoron. Uranus, the planet of sudden upheaval, is all about change, while Taurus is notorious for resisting it. And no offense to Taurus, but they are incredibly slow to do much of anything, preferring instead to fall into the predictability of routine. Thus with Uranus in Taurus, there is a journey around having to grapple with what *needs* to change, even if you don't like it or want it. The flip side of this is that the changes Uranus does bring about tend to stick. The avenues of pleasure, resources, and embracing your sensual nature can bring about incredible liberation.

What to Try in the Bedroom

+ Slow sex—go longer than you normally do or see just how long you can last until you're spent.
+ Introduce food into the bedroom or during foreplay.
+ Focus on the throat as an erogenous zone.
+ Integrate sensual experiences into sex, such as something that engages all five senses.
+ Alternatively, try sensory deprivation, such as a blindfold.

URANUS IN GEMINI

Uranus finds itself in an interesting position in Mercury-ruled Gemini, as Uranus is the higher octave of Mercury—meaning Uranus takes all the characteristics of the planet of communication and elevates or expands upon them. Certainly the themes of communication, learning, and travel can act as catalysts for great change. The need to be flexible, curious, and open to new ways of doing things is paramount. Remember that Gemini is the sign that's best at putting themselves in another person's shoes and understanding varying thoughts and feelings. With Uranus in Gemini, there is much to be gained from open and honest connections, as well as following the many threads of interest here.

What to Try in the Bedroom

+ Dirty talk, playing switch, or just embracing and cultivating more versatility in your sexual expression.
+ Try the opposite approach to the way you normally do things.
+ Use your hands more during foreplay and sex.
+ Bring someone else into the bedroom with you and your partner just for fun (assuming everyone is down!).

URANUS IN CANCER

With Uranus in Cancer, change comes through the avenue of nurturing. The family of origin and everything that entails may be a source of great upheaval for you. The home may be, too. You may move a lot throughout your lifetime and/or experience some kind of instability in those areas. With this placement, finding a safe and stable place to lay your head, as well as getting your emotional needs met, can offer radical change but in a more fulfilling way. Having your own family and taking on the role of parent can too.

What to Try in the Bedroom

+ Show off your chest and/or stomach; focus on these areas as erogenous zones.
+ Try playing the submissive role.
+ Bring more playfulness into the bedroom.
+ Open yourself up to a deep emotional and spiritual connection with your partner.
+ Lovemaking over fucking.

URANUS IN LEO

Again we see an emphasis on the need for authenticity and self-expression with Uranus in Leo. Embodying all your unique gifts in a bold and passionate way will open the doors to liberation. Creativity is a huge focus for Uranus here, which pushes you to share your creative visions and unique perspectives. Therefore, having a hobby or two through which to channel all your creative potential is important. Embracing your dramatic, charismatic, and warmhearted nature will set you free.

What to Try in the Bedroom

+ Being absolutely worshiped and/or begging for it.
+ Giving and receiving back massages.
+ Self-pleasure.
+ Being bold and dramatic in your sexual expression.

+ Hair-pulling.
+ Passionate lovemaking.

URANUS IN VIRGO

Similar to what we see with this planet in Gemini, Uranus is again in an interesting spot when in the second Mercury-ruled sign of Virgo. Communication again comes forward to open the doors to freedom, though the communication style here is sharp, keen, and discerning. With Uranus in Virgo, developing systems to help with organization and simplification is somehow important, as is a focus on good health practices. Freeing yourself from the pitfalls of perfectionism and a harsh inner critic will bring about the change you're looking for.

What to Try in the Bedroom

+ Sleeping with someone older or more experienced.
+ Letting your partner lead/top.
+ Being tied up/light BDSM.
+ Mutual oral sex.
+ Incorporating toys in the bedroom.
+ Crotchless underwear.
+ Voyeurism.

URANUS IN LIBRA

With Uranus in Libra, relationships act as the catalyst for radical change. The Uranian influence manifests as an unconventional approach to love. This is yet another placement in the chart that can point to things like polyamory or other more experimental forms of romance. If nothing else, you are attracted to truly unique people who likely stand out or break the mold in some way.

On top of this, something about the experiences you have in your love life can be both ungrounding and liberating. Across your lifetime, you may experience both extremes: great unrest and great satisfaction. At some point there is a need to find true balance in your life in order to curb the dramatic ups and downs of Uranus. With this planet in Libra, there may also be a need to find justice for yourself in some way.

What to Try in the Bedroom

+ Sixty-nine or any kind of mutual play.
+ Ass play.
+ Dressing to show off the lower back or highlighting the butt in some way.
+ Licking.
+ Mirror play.
+ Nipple play.
+ Inverted sexual positions.
+ Teasing and/or edging.

URANUS IN SCORPIO

In sultry Scorpio, we see Uranus manifest through sex, period. You seek to find radical change, liberation, and transformation through the pleasures of the flesh. This likely manifests through some sort of kink (or three) and encourages exploration and reframing around what others might consider taboo or perverse in some way. With Uranus in Scorpio, there's a need to break through the boundaries of intimacy and sexuality and explore new ways of expressing your erotic nature. Power dynamics usually play a big role here.

What to Try in the Bedroom

+ Anal and/or ass play.
+ Mutual worship/obsession.
+ Anything involving control and power dynamics.
+ Leather and latex.
+ Collars.
+ Any kind of exploration around BDSM and kink.
+ Passionate lovemaking.

URANUS IN SAGITTARIUS

The planet of experimentation finds a certain kinship with exploratory Sagittarius, who seeks to experience as many different things as they can in life. The types of experiences that you seek out may vary greatly or seem unusual in some way. Anything new or unique or something that only a few people have done appeals greatly to you. With Uranus in Sagittarius, being able to honor your sense of adventure and embracing the daredevil within can be highly transformative. Radical change can also come through travel, spirituality, and religion or maybe even through the experiences gained while pursuing higher education.

What to Try in the Bedroom

+ Sleeping with a stranger.
+ Anything that feels adventurous and fun.
+ Dressing to highlight the thighs and/or hips.
+ Exhibitionism.
+ Sleeping with someone while traveling.
+ Striptease.
+ Having multiple partners and/or group sex.

URANUS IN CAPRICORN

Uranus in traditional Capricorn is a bit of an oxymoron. You ultimately are here to challenge or push the boundaries of the status quo in some way, but not in the same way we see with this planet in Aquarius. Ultimately, Uranus in Capricorn is about challenging tradition. What's still working? What isn't? Who is in power and what is the extent of their influence? Capricorn is all about integrity and living their values, and Uranus shows up to kick down the door of tradition, to force you to break free from long-standing values that limit you in order to live a life more in alignment with what you truly stand for. These traditions can be both familial and societal. But at some point, you are going to have to assess what *you* stand for, regardless of what has been taught to you, in order to find true liberation and freedom.

What to Try in the Bedroom

- Domination.
- Wearing leather, corsets, or anything super structural or binding.
- Spanking.
- BDSM.
- Shibari.
- Garters and lingerie.
- Power dynamics.
- Extended foreplay.
- Wearing a uniform or sleeping with someone in uniform.

URANUS IN AQUARIUS

In Aquarius, we find Uranus in its only home, as the modern-day ruler of the water bearer. In that sense, whenever we speak about the planet or the sign, we are basically saying the same thing. The Uranian themes of technology, innovation, equality, humanitarianism, and freedom shine brightly through the Aquarian lens, as the energy of Uranus is able to show up in its purest form here.

With Uranus in Aquarius, you are ready to rebel and shatter the ceiling on anything corrupt and to break down the systems in society that stand in the way of true community and advancement. Truly, you are here to push the conversation of humanity forward in some way, which may simply boil down to being your most radical, authentic self in a society that would seek to silence you. Authenticity is an act of rebellion and liberates not only you but also those around you.

What to Try in the Bedroom

- Phone or cybersex.
- Group sex and/or sex clubs.
- Anything that feels totally different from what you normally do in bed.
- Restraints, cages, or sex swings.
- Costumes.
- Pantyhose, fishnets, garters.

URANUS IN PISCES

In the final sign of the zodiac, Uranus shines through the Piscean themes of spirituality, compassion, the arts, and mental health. With Uranus in Pisces, you are ready to break through conventional approaches to mental health as well as their accompanying stigmas. The unlimited compassion and understanding of Pisces becomes the catalyst for change and somehow ends up changing everything for you. Expressing yourself creatively, acting in service to others, spirituality, and religion are all avenues to greater freedom in your life, as is embracing your dreams—both nighttime dreams and personal aspirations.

What to Try in the Bedroom

+ Submission.
+ Any and all of your fantasies (and your partner's!).
+ Role-play.
+ A foot massage or feet play.
+ Wearing rubber, latex, and sexy shoes.
+ Cuckolding.
+ Slow, tender sex.

A NOTE ON HOUSES

To better understand the nature of your Uranus placement, it's important to explore the house it resides in within your birth chart. The area of life that the respective house rules over points to where and how we experience the shocking nature of Uranian events. I think it's important to understand that most of the time Uranus is pretty dormant. We only experience Uranus every now and again, usually when it's activated by a transit, for example. However, there is no confusing when we *do* experience Uranus, as it's always shocking and unexpected and comes seemingly out of nowhere. These events, while fleeting, upend pretty much everything, and therefore change everything overnight as well. While the unexpected nature of Uranus makes it difficult to predict how these events will manifest, the house Uranus is in points to the area of our lives where we experience these extreme events time and again. For example, Uranus in the ninth house may show up as unexpected travel or unexpected events during travel that completely change our perspective. Uranus in the fourth house may be suddenly needing to move for some reason. Uranus in the fifth house may be a surprise pregnancy or a whirlwind romance, and so on.

Beyond this, the house with Uranus in it also points to the area of our lives where we are different from those around us. Remember that Uranus is also about our inner genius! This house shows where and how our visionary powers can come through and shine and also where we may be ahead of the curve in some way. Uranus in the third house is a great example. As the house of writing, learning, and the student, Uranus here denotes someone who is incredibly smart and may be able to see things or understand things about a certain topic that is innovative or novel in some way. Einstein had Uranus in the third house and he was a literal genius, and the implications of his work still have a profound impact on science today. Read up on the house your Uranus is in to see where your inner genius is begging to come out and play.

9

NEPTUNE ♆

MODERN-DAY RULER OF: Pisces

HIGHER OCTAVE OF: Venus

Neptune is a particularly interesting planet to consider within the realm of sextrology. Its energy is especially elusive, slippery, and difficult to define. The nature of Neptune is hazy, dreamy, and romantic, ruling over things like the imagination, escapism, addiction, drugs, creativity, spirituality, and all things fantasy. On the one hand, this fog can feel romantic and hazy, as if we're walking around with a set of rose-tinted glasses on, making everything feel warm, fuzzy, and honey-drenched. As the higher octave of Venus, Neptune expands on and elevates all the Venusian indulgences of the heart and the flesh. Both these planets strive to achieve the higher ideals of humanity. Venus does this through the pursuit of beauty and personal, intimate love, while Neptune expands these ideals through unconditional love and spiritual connection. Utopian Neptune views love, romance, aesthetics, and the arts as spiritual necessities, elevating the ideals of Venus to impossible heights. This is why Venus is exalted in Pisces, the sign that is Neptune's natural home.

On the other hand, though, Neptune can also create illusion and delusion, eclipsing mental clarity and making it difficult to pin down what's real and what's not when it comes to relationships. In this way, we must be careful to maintain healthy boundaries and make sure we haven't idealized someone to the point that we've become lost to reality. No matter what, though, in sextrology we channel the dreamy nature of Neptune through our sexual fantasies.

Because it takes Neptune 165 years to make its way around the Sun—and therefore through the entire zodiacal wheel—there has never been a time when the people living on Earth have had Neptune placements that span all twelve signs.

NEPTUNE IN ARIES

With Neptune in Aries, we see a combination of the idealism and spirituality of Neptune and the boldness and initiative of the cosmic ram, resulting in individuals who are both visionary and action-oriented, with a strong sense of purpose and a willingness to challenge the status quo.

NEPTUNE IN TAURUS

With Neptune in earthy Taurus, the themes of resources, stability, and pleasure come to the forefront to hold hands with fantasy and idealism. This is an especially indulgent position of Neptune, describing individuals who strive for a life full of fleshy, sensual pleasure.

NEPTUNE IN GEMINI

When Neptune is in Gemini, we see individuals who dream about a world full of free-flowing communication, information, and possibilities. Because Gemini has a finger in virtually every pie, these lovers know that variety is truly the spice of life. They are open to all kinds of perspectives, values, and ways of doing things and are constantly on the hunt for something new.

NEPTUNE IN CANCER

In a way, Neptune thrives in Cancer. The nurturing, intuitive, caring, and spiritual ideals of Cancer blend quite nicely with the motivations of Neptune, which are almost exactly the same, creating a certain ease of expression with this placement.

NEPTUNE IN LEO

In bold and creative Leo, Neptune is quite heart-centered. The warmth, charisma, and generosity of Leo gets channeled through the rose-colored lens of Neptune, elevating the self-expression that Leo craves. This is actually a super creative position of Neptune, as Leo is also prone to fantasies and thrives on creativity and drama.

NEPTUNE IN VIRGO

When Neptune is in Virgo, we see the ideals of Neptune blended with themes of service, health, and work systems. While these individuals are certainly motivated by helping others, there is an extra high propensity for sacrifice here, so much so that they may take on too much, ultimately to their detriment. Burnout is a real possibility, which can then start to affect their health, as there is an innate connection here between spiritual and physical health. Remember that Neptune makes us more susceptible to things, and in the case of people with Neptune in Virgo, striving for perfection can create unrealistic expectations that end up affecting their health.

The flip side of this is that Neptune in Virgo grants these individuals a psychic connection to their body, and when they are dialed in, they will always know what's going on with their physical vessel and health. It also means they respond strongly to substances, which can be both good and bad.

NEPTUNE IN LIBRA

Those with their Neptune in Libra want to see life and the world as a fair place to be. They believe that true peace and harmony could be attained if only people would treat each other fairly and justly. Cooperation and seeing and hearing all sides of the story are what these people are good at, as it's only fair to do so. They prefer not to judge others, but instead look to find compromise in their connections. Certainly relationships in general are the focus here, as Libra is the sign of partnership.

Indeed, people with Neptune in Libra love love and tend to idealize their partners. They are romantic and like to get swept up in the rosy haze of love.

The dreamy fog of Neptune can cloud their ability to see their lovers clearly, and because of that, they are susceptible to tolerating bad behavior and putting more of themselves into a relationship than the other person. Boundaries are especially important here, as is making sure they see people for who they really are.

NEPTUNE IN SCORPIO

With Neptune in deep and intense Scorpio, we see the intuitive powers of the scorpion blended with the psychic faculties of Neptune, which creates a powerful combo of gifts for these lovers. Unlike those with their Neptune in Libra, the Neptune in Scorpio generation doesn't necessarily believe in fairness and equality, instead preferring to feel people out individually and intuit what is best based upon what they learn. Scorpio knows better than most that circumstances have a huge effect on people, and to ignore someone's subjective experiences and influences would do them a disservice.

Because Scorpio grapples greatly with power and control, these lovers may struggle with these issues throughout their lives. This can manifest as a need for control, a lack of control, or not seeing power dynamics between themselves and others clearly. Over the course of a lifetime, all that may be true.

Beyond this, Neptune in Scorpio individuals are likely to idealize sex, pleasure, and eroticism as a whole. They may in fact use sex as a means to escape all the harshness of reality, using its transformative powers like a drug.

NEPTUNE IN SAGITTARIUS

Those with their Neptune in Sagittarius are optimistic as hell. They have a strong vision when it comes to an ideal world, which centers around freedom, religion and spirituality, and lots and lots of adventure. Similar to Neptune in Scorpio, Neptune in Sagittarius is a powerful spiritual placement, as both the planet and the sign value walking the spiritual path and experiencing union with the Divine.

While the optimism of Neptune in Sagittarius can be refreshing, these individuals have to be careful to make sure their positive mindset isn't impeding their ability to live in reality and see things the way they really are. In my opinion, this is where we can see the insidious "positive vibes only" mentality take root, which encourages spiritual bypassing and discourages actually dealing with the full spectrum of what it means to be human.

The other thing to watch out for with this placement is the religious fanatic or zealot. Cults fall in the domain of both Neptune and Sagittarius, so this combo may make a person especially vulnerable to being swept up by such things. Because New Age spirituality and, honestly, spirituality and religion as a whole cultivate environments that make it all too easy to get lost in the sauce, it's important for these individuals to keep their feet on the ground and take their time discerning what is truth and what is pure fiction.

NEPTUNE IN CAPRICORN

In traditional and wise Capricorn, Neptune manifests quite differently than in many other signs. Thanks to the especially grounded, logical, and realistic nature of Capricorn, individuals with this placement don't struggle with the delusional nature of Neptune as much as other groups do. Their fantasies tend to be rooted in reality, with Capricorn's influence commanding a pragmatism that aids in discerning what is achievable and realistic and what is not.

That said, there can be a cynical and/or pessimistic streak to Neptune in Capricorn, as faith and fantasy aren't really motivators here. In that sense, Neptune's influence begins to show its face through a cynicism that may not be warranted or a depression that inhibits the ability to see things clearly. While these individuals are the most able to turn their dreams into reality, there is a lack of imagination and inspiration here that must be overcome.

NEPTUNE IN AQUARIUS

Those with their Neptune in Aquarius are humanitarians. Their ideals center around creating a world that is equal, accessible, and sustainable for everyone regardless of religion, race, gender, sexuality, social and economic class, etc. They value both individuality and the collective and strive for ultimate freedom.

Certainly these individuals are open-minded. They are ready to learn and explore all things, though this is also the generation that is the most prone to using technology as a means of escape. Doomscrolling on social media, anyone?

Alternatively, when we blend the innovative nature of Aquarius with the idealistic, imaginative nature of Neptune, we see a group of people who are likely to push the boundaries of what is possible via science and technology. AI might be a great example of this. As we move more and more toward becoming a technology-dependent society, it should be interesting to see what these folks end up doing for humanity.

These folks are the most idealistic of the Neptunian bunch.

NEPTUNE IN PISCES

As the modern-day ruler of Pisces, Neptune is very much considered to be at home in the final sign of the zodiac. Similar to Uranus in Aquarius, Neptune in Pisces is a placement where the planet and the sign are essentially saying the same thing twice.

The beauty of Neptune in Pisces is that it places an emphasis on creativity, beauty, love, spirituality, empathy, and compassion. This is an especially sensitive placement of Neptune, and at its best, it elevates all the wonderful potential of this planet. These individuals are idealistic and have a vivid imagination, with the creative prowess to become prolific artists and creatives.

However, I would be remiss not to mention the escapist potential that is particularly strong here. Having Neptune at home in Pisces heightens the aversion to the harsh realities of life that this sign is known for, and these individuals are especially prone to the self-destructive tendencies that can result. Because Pisces rules over drugs and addiction and because Neptune increases our sensitivity to substances, it's important for these folks to be especially aware and safe should they wish to experiment or party.

A NOTE ON HOUSES

Beyond the sign that Neptune is in, we also have to look to the house it resides in. The themes of that house play an important twofold role. First, we see an area of our lives where we may struggle to see things clearly or be seen clearly. For example, those with Neptune in the first house often have qualities or fantasies projected onto them by other people. They may also struggle to see themselves clearly. Someone with Neptune in the seventh house may struggle to see their partners clearly and may look at their relationships through rose-tinted glasses, for better or worse. Those with Neptune in the fourth house may struggle to understand the reality of their family issues or dynamics or struggle to see their mother clearly, and so on.

The second dynamic of Neptune in any given house describes where we seek refuge and escape from the harshness of the world. With Neptune in the fourth house, the person's home may be their refuge or oasis away from everyone and everything, or perhaps they find comfort in spending time with their family. Someone with Neptune in the eleventh house may seek comfort through friends or scrolling away on social media.

To better understand your own Neptune placement, read the relevant house description in the chapter on houses (chapter 17).

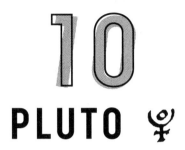

PLUTO ♇

MODERN-DAY RULER OF: Scorpio

HIGHER OCTAVE OF: Mars

As the final planet in the chart and the one farthest from the Sun in our solar system, Pluto moves through the signs the slowest. Because of that, Pluto ends up with the largest "generations" of people contained within one sign—larger than those of any other planet or point in the chart. Pluto, unlike the other planets, doesn't have a fixed time period that it spends in any given sign, thanks to its elliptical orbit of the Sun, which is more of an oval shape than a true circle. This unique characteristic has Pluto spending anywhere from twelve to thirty years in one sign, spending the most amount of time in Taurus and the least in Scorpio, its home sign.

Thanks to this special categorization, Pluto's influence in sextrology is unlike anything else. Pluto is the higher octave of Mars. Much like Uranus and Neptune, Pluto takes all the Martian ideals and expands them to the extremes, including sex, magnetizing it in a way that only the outermost planet can. Within the bounds of sextrology, Pluto plays a powerful role, representing the ideals of power and control, sex, destruction and creation, cycles of death and rebirth, deep healing, and, ultimately, transformation.

It's important to understand that Pluto is deeply karmic in nature as well. Wherever it sits in the chart represents themes that we will return to time and again, in perpetuity, during our entire lives. In sextrology this is no exception. The cyclical nature of Pluto plays out time and again as we seek to find empowerment in Pluto's arena—especially if Pluto is in close contact with any other planet, especially one of the partnership planets or points.

Because it takes Pluto about 250 years to make its way around the Sun, there will never be a point in time when the people living on Earth have Pluto in all twelve signs. I will be focusing here on Pluto in the houses rather than the signs, as well as Pluto in aspect to the planets and points covered in this book.

PLUTO AND THE SUN

Whenever we see Pluto in aspect to the Sun, there is a lifelong karmic journey around the identity. Especially if Pluto is conjunct the Sun, this is someone who may feel they are constantly engaged in the cycles of life, death, and rebirth when it comes to who they are. They've likely experienced a number of events in their life that have completely shattered their notion of self and have had to evolve in order to rebuild. Pluto also brings an undeniable intensity to anyone with this dynamic in their chart.

As is the true Plutonian way, these lovers will always come back to the journey of self-discovery to some extent, having to peel back the layers of who they are time and again, relentlessly shedding the dead weight of old identities that no longer serve or resonate. More than for any other Plutonian dynamic in the chart, the exploration and knowledge of the self is the most important for those with Pluto in aspect to their Sun. Learning how to express themselves in an authentic way will open the door to empowerment and transformation. This is also true when it comes to their sexual identity. Learning how to embody erotic energy in a genuine way—whatever that may mean—can act as a powerful catalyst.

PLUTO AND THE MOON

With Pluto aspecting the other luminary in the chart, the journey shifts from the identity to the emotions. Moon-Pluto aspects create an unfathomably deep feeler who likely struggles when grappling with the extreme intensity of their own feelings. Inside they likely experience a great amount of tumult around their emotions, seeming to feel things more deeply than those around them, and indeed that's probably true.

It's difficult to overstate the depth of emotion these lovers possess. Regardless of the sign the Moon sits in, their feelings are extremely intense, even, say, in a normally levelheaded earth sign. They may struggle to deal with the power of their feelings and may also grapple with lots of emotional pain throughout their lives.

For those with a Moon-Pluto aspect, there may also be literal issues with the mother and/or the family of origin in general. Certainly their emotional needs were not met as a child, for whatever reason. They may come from an emotionally abusive or neglectful family as well.

No matter what the situation may be, it is through emotional healing that real transformation occurs for these individuals. Therapy and other supportive means are something they should consider, as well as developing strong boundaries to help protect themselves.

PLUTO AND MERCURY

When Pluto shows up to influence the journey of Mercury, the path to transformation surrounds communication, specifically around speaking up and sharing one's thoughts, feelings, knowledge, and perspective.

With Mercury-Pluto aspects, communication can be a difficult, fickle thing. Even though it's one of the most important things when it comes to any and all kinds of relationships, I think we all struggle with it from time to time. However, for these individuals it may feel especially difficult. They may have experienced being silenced in their lives or had experiences that showed them that what they have to say isn't valuable, and so on. Despite this, however, it is only through finding the power in their voice that real empowerment can happen. In that sense, there may be a need to push back against fear and/or those who don't seem to value what they have to say by speaking their truth anyway. Once these lovers are able to do so, they will find that they begin to attract more fulfilling experiences and connections.

PLUTO AND VENUS

When Pluto is connected to Venus in the birth chart, the karmic evolution of the Lord of the Underworld plays out through romantic relationships.

As somebody who has Venus conjunct Pluto in my own chart, I can tell you that this is not an easy journey. While Pluto brings an insane amount of passion and intensity to romance, it also brings just as much pain. Unfortunately, at least in the beginning, all of us with Venus-Pluto aspects will have to grapple with some serious bullshit. Things like abuse, cheating, trauma, and the like are all too common for people with this dynamic in the chart. Power and control come to the forefront in their relationships, which can manifest both within their partners and within their own self. It may take a great deal of time to get over a painful relationship, if it can be done at all.

However, because romantic relationships will always be the avenue through which transformation occurs, all hope is not lost. Through shedding the layers of unhealthy habits and connections, these individuals can begin to find transformation and healing through the joy and beauty of love instead of the painful lessons.

I would also like to note that there is something about the way any person with Venus-Pluto in their chart loves that is transformative.

PLUTO AND MARS

There is no other dynamic in astrology that points more overtly to a journey around sex as a whole than Mars-Pluto aspects. Pluto turns its transformative sights on its lower octave, Mars, and brings the question of sex to the forefront. Especially if Pluto is conjunct the red planet, we see an almost impossibly high sex drive. There is a voraciousness and an insatiability to the sexual appetite of these lovers. Their passion runs just as deep as their hunger, and there is an incredible need to express that desire in a physical way. However, it's important to remember that even with a powerful sex drive, these individuals still have to grapple with the transformative journey of Pluto over the course of their lives. Pluto comes in to ask, What does healthy sexuality look like? What does it mean to truly be empowered in your erotic nature? These questions will be circled back to time and again. As these individuals grow, evolve, and change throughout their lives, their sexual energy will do the same.

Outside of sex, there is, inevitably, also a journey around anger and action for these lovers. More than for any other Plutonian journey, these individuals will also have to grapple with their powerful anger, both how to have a healthy relationship with it and how to express it in a healthy way. Moving the body as a way to channel all their pent-up energy is a great place to start.

PLUTO AND JUPITER

In a way, having Pluto and Jupiter aspecting each other in the natal chart can be quite nice. For these individuals, the Greater Benefic's themes of expansion, abundance, and good fortune act as the avenue to powerful growth and transformation—not too shabby! Certainly there is great potential to be unlocked through truly understanding the nature of their Jupiter placement and how to embody that energy in order to attract Jupiter's promise of fortune—which, when paired with the intensity of Pluto, creates an environment for an extreme amount of expansion.

However, I would not be fulfilling my duties as an astrologer if I didn't include the caveat that we don't truly know what Jupiter is going to expand. Because of this, it *is* important to have some discernment and boundaries here. Too much of a good thing really can transform into a bad thing. With the extremes that Pluto operates under, we need to be careful what we wish for!

Beyond that, Jupiterian avenues such as spirituality, travel, knowledge, and optimism show up as agents of change for people with Jupiter-Pluto aspects. Embracing the qualities of their Jupiter in relationships (as described in the Jupiter chapter) becomes even more important.

PLUTO AND SATURN

Saturn-Pluto aspects in the chart bring together the themes of power and authority in a real way. I'll be honest and say this dynamic in the chart can feel particularly difficult, considering the energies of Saturn are often difficult for people anyway, as we are forced to grapple with limitations, obstacles, and the incredibly slow nature of Saturn that plays out over exceedingly long periods of time.

However, something I invite you all to consider is that before the inception of modern and evolutionary astrology, Saturn ruled as the final planet in the solar system for a long time (hence its association with boundaries, as it was believed to mark the very boundary of existence!). Before the discovery of Pluto, many of the qualities we now associate with the Lord of the Underworld were ascribed to Saturn. Therefore, Pluto and Saturn actually work quite well together, as they're ultimately asking us for the same things in a lot of ways.

When it comes to sextrology, Saturn-Pluto aspects require us to dismantle the traditions and values that we've been indoctrinated into one way or another—or, at the very least, we have to have an honest look at them. What messages about sex were we given growing up? Are they constricting, limiting, or outdated in some way? What kinds of foundations do we need to lay around our values and integrity when it comes to sex? And so on.

Keep in mind that working with Saturn effectively requires a certain amount of experience that can only come with time.

PLUTO AND URANUS

The combination of Pluto and Uranus is pretty unique. Because Uranus can feel dormant most of the time and then suddenly rear its head with little to no warning, this dynamic in the birth chart creates shocking and/or unexpected moments that act as a catalyst for change and evolution. The very nature of Uranian events seems to change everything overnight, often leading to a total overhaul in some way. With Pluto's influence in the mix, the transformative powers of both planets combine to supercharge the influence of Uranus. Keep in mind, too, that Uranus rules over the higher mind and represents the inner genius in each of us. Therefore, this can be a powerful combo for the intellect as well as for spirituality. Because Uranus rules over all things unique and ahead of its time, there's something about embracing the visionary aspects of ourselves that can act as an impressive means of evolution as well.

From a sexual perspective, exploring new things in relationships can open up our horizons and help us to get more in touch with our authenticity.

PLUTO AND NEPTUNE

Neptune-Pluto combinations in the chart are exceedingly rare. In fact, because the cycle of Pluto and Neptune plays out ultimately over a 500-year period, this is the rarest combination a person can have in the birth chart, especially if Neptune and Pluto are conjunct. In fact, the last time these two planets were conjunct was back in the 1890s, and the next time they will meet up won't be until the 2380s. However, there are plenty of other aspects that can be made between these two other than the conjunction.

I will say that of all the possible combinations a chart can have with Pluto, the ones concerning Neptune are the most inherently spiritual. At its core, Neptune represents spirituality and our connection to all things ethereal and otherworldly. When Pluto joins the conversation, there's something about the spiritual journey that becomes important for these individuals. Embracing their gifts, fantasies, and creativity can act as the stage for empowerment and transformation. Exploring the power of their imagination and allowing it to express itself fully can be key. These themes extend to sextrology as well, inviting play into the bedroom as a means of empowerment. There's something about the whimsy and softness of this combination that might surprise you.

PLUTO IN THE FIRST HOUSE

Pluto brings an undeniable intensity to anybody with the venerable Lord of the Underworld in the first house, similar to what we see when Pluto is in tight conjunction with the Sun. These individuals openly embody all the traits of Pluto, for better or worse, and in that sense are fundamentally Plutonian. They may grapple with any number of things, including issues of control, mistrust, power struggles, and the like. Ultimately the journey surrounds the identity and the search to feel empowered in who they are. Again we see a lifelong, perpetual cycle of life, death, and rebirth here. They may also struggle to connect with people, as there will inevitably be those who shy away from the Pluto person's intense nature, especially because the Pluto person will demand an unrelenting intensity from others, too. More than for any other position of Pluto, these lovers aren't interested in any kind of shallow or vapid connection. They thrive on diving almost impossibly deep into the human condition, and those who aren't ready to have themselves revealed will find the Pluto person's piercing perceptions to be unnerving. However, if this happens to be your own natal placement, I highly encourage you to make peace with this, since you'd never be satisfied having relationships with those who can't match your depth anyway.

Beyond this, Pluto in the first house imparts an incredible sexual, animal magnetism to the aura that is both alluring and intimidating. People are drawn to a first house Pluto, though they may not always know why. Something about the energy they embody acts as a catalyst for transformation in those they come in contact with.

Your Plutonian Superpower

Pluto in the first house gives you an incredible amount of personal power, arguably more than any other position of Pluto in the chart. Your ability to move through anything and everything that comes your way in life, transforming that energy into even more power, makes you capable of a great deal. It also ups your personal magnetism and allure. You are capable of attracting who and what you want into your orbit. In a way you are undefeatable, and it's simply a matter of remembering this that enables you to overcome and thrive.

Pluto in the first house also gives you a piercing perception into the true nature of those around you. Your intuition is formidable, too. With great power comes great responsibility.

PLUTO IN THE SECOND HOUSE

For those with Pluto in the second house, there exists a lifelong journey around financial and material security as well as self-worth and pleasure. There are any number of ways this can manifest, of course, but some examples include growing up in a situation that didn't feel safe one way or another, especially with money playing a key role in that; money being used as a means of control in some way; or experiencing financial extremes, such as going from having a lot of money to suddenly having none. As these individuals become adults, they may struggle to figure out how to provide themselves with the correct resources and money to cultivate any kind of security and safety in a tangible way.

The journey for those with Pluto in the second house fuses together the themes of resources and self-confidence. These people must find a way to trust their ability to be resourceful, to reach down into themselves and find the tools they need to handle whatever is thrown their way. Keep in mind that this isn't limited to just money. Once they're able to trust themselves to be able to provide for and take care of themselves, their self-esteem solidifies as well. The trick is to find and cultivate a feeling of stability within themselves, regardless of their financial situation. When one becomes rooted, so, too, does the other. It's a symbiotic relationship. Iron sharpens iron.

Your Plutonian Superpower

In the second house, Pluto makes you extremely resourceful. When you put your mind to it, you are able to secure anything and everything you need to solve whatever problems arise in life. When you can learn to trust yourself in this way, the power of Pluto unlocks and makes itself available to you.

On a more mundane level, Pluto in the second house gives you an intuitive sense about money and values. You have a sharp instinct around what is actually worth it, literally and figuratively, and you are likely quite good at managing money and resources, both yours and other people's.

An interesting fact when it comes to Pluto in the second house is that many billionaires, such as Bill Gates, have this placement in their chart. This is one example of how Pluto operates in extremes and takes us from famine to feast. Now, this doesn't mean everyone with this placement will become a billionaire, but it does demonstrate your capability to generate wealth, however you define it, for yourself.

PLUTO IN THE THIRD HOUSE

In the third house, the Plutonian journey surrounds communication, similar to what we see when Pluto aspects Mercury. These individuals may struggle to speak up, to share what they think, know, and feel, and they certainly struggle to feel heard by those around them. In fact, they may feel they're excellent communicators, but for whatever reason, no matter how hard they try, their words seem to perpetually fall on deaf ears.

Because the third is the house of the local community as well as siblings, for these individuals there may also be a karmic journey with siblings, should they have any, as well as the town they grew up in. For whatever reason, there exists a fundamental mismatch between the Pluto person and the people immediately around them. Oftentimes the call here is to leave their hometown and venture out into the world. By doing so, they are more apt to find the right relationships where they feel seen, heard, and accepted.

Your Plutonian Superpower

When Pluto resides in the third house, we see somebody with a voracious appetite for knowledge and an investigative mind. These lovers are able to cut through to the meat of any subject and uncover information that others may not even be aware of. They are excellent students who have a lot to offer. Because of this, they are able to bring about powerful transformation to those in their immediate surroundings. They may be quite active in their local environment and/or go on frequent short-term trips that act as a catalyst for change.

PLUTO IN THE FOURTH HOUSE

Similar to Moon-Pluto aspects, Pluto in the fourth house can indicate a difficult upbringing—which may be putting it lightly. There exists a deep wound within the family of origin that can manifest any number of ways. And no matter what that reason may be, growing up wasn't a safe or healthy situation. Maybe they grew up in an abusive household; maybe their parents were addicts; maybe they were taken away from their parents. The list of possibilities is long. In my experience, this position of Pluto tends to manifest especially in the person's relationship with their mother—though, again, not always. No matter what the circumstance may be, healing comes through establishing their own family, whether that's the family they build through marriage and children, through friends, or both.

For those with Pluto in the fourth house, ideally there is also healing to be had with their family of origin, likely through plenty of self-work, therapy, boundaries, and defining what a healthy, sustainable relationship with them means to the Pluto person. In my opinion, this is a highly subjective journey.

Your Plutonian Superpower

As much as those with Pluto in the fourth house may feel like the black sheep of the family, they are the ones who are here to bring change to their bloodline. Oftentimes in spiritual circles we hear about people who are generational curse breakers; that title was made with this placement in mind.

As frustrating as it may feel, these babes are here to cut off the unhealthy cycles that exist within their family in favor of something better. Through their very existence they are transforming the pain of their ancestors into something greater. They are the ones showing their family the way to greater love and better practices in relationships.

PLUTO IN THE FIFTH HOUSE

Pluto in the fifth house grapples with the idea of joy, romance, and creativity as a means of transformation. In a way, the intensity of Pluto in the fifth house can feel deeply at odds with the lighthearted nature of this house. It's likely that these lovers struggle with the concept of fun—they may not even know what the word "fun" really means to them.

In my opinion, a big lesson for those with Pluto in the fifth house is that not everything is that deep. I can feel the immediate protestations of these Plutonians now, but it's true. Sometimes doing things simply because we want to, because it sounds like a good time, is reason enough, and embracing that philosophy is actually quite powerful for these lovers. As counterintuitive as it may seem, learning to lighten up will unlock the doors to evolution for these lovers, especially because pleasure is likely something that was robbed from them and their lives from an early age.

Speaking of childhood, those with Pluto in the fifth house probably didn't have an easy one. For whatever reason, things may have been hard as a kid. Something about the circumstances they grew up in didn't provide what they needed to be able to just play and be a kid. Therefore, channeling the idea of fun through the lens of long-lost childhood interests would be fantastic as well. Truly the goal is authentic self-expression, whatever that means to them, even if it's silly as hell. Having a creative hobby is one of the best things for those with Pluto in the fifth, as is learning how to live in the moment and be present here and now. Children may also play a role in transformation for these people, whether through interacting with them, having their own, or both.

Beyond that, romance also plays a big role for individuals with Pluto in the fifth house. Through the Plutonian lens, the call is to learn and experience new forms of love that weave in self-love, acceptance, and joy.

Your Plutonian Superpower

In the fifth house, Pluto grants a potent creativity. Through whichever mediums they choose, these lovers are able to communicate all the complexities of being human, laying bare not only their own truths but also the grander truths of the human condition.

When they are given room to breathe, the works they produce enable them to express themselves in a way they truly need, leading to healing, transformation, and empowerment. They find joy in allowing their inner child to come to the surface and play. In fact, they may be better at this than the rest of us!

PLUTO IN THE SIXTH HOUSE

Personally I find the sixth house to be a curious place for Pluto in the chart. As the sixth is the most mundane of the houses, ruling over the ins and outs of our day-to-day lives, the intensity of Pluto plays out in a very different way here than in other areas of the natal chart. What I mean when I say this is that the journey for those with Pluto in the sixth house depends greatly on the circumstances and is highly individual.

On the one hand, figuring out how to adult through developing a daily routine may be the focus for those with Pluto in the sixth house, and it may be something they struggle to establish in a real way. There's something about the experiences they have in their daily lives that may feel intense and/or difficult in some way likely *because* they have experienced an incredible amount of change in the course of their lives. Finding a way to establish stability through routines can become an incredible grounding force that offers them the structure they need to thrive.

On the other hand, Pluto can have a profound impact on a person's health. In my experience with clients, people with this position of Pluto can have extreme health issues—though not always. I have known people who are constantly dealing with serious, chronic health issues that are never-ending, and I've known people with this placement who haven't dealt with much at all. Again, Pluto operates in the extremes, so we tend to fall on one end of the spectrum or the other. Regardless, for those with Pluto in the sixth house, more than for any other placement of this planet in the chart, there is a need to prioritize health and take care of their physical vessel. Having a body that feels good also offers them the grounding and stability they need to thrive.

Your Plutonian Superpower

Because of the connection to the physical body with the sixth house, those with Pluto here make incredible healthcare providers. They have an intuitive connection to the body that can help get to the root of an underlying issue that may evade detection. Regardless of whether or not they actually go into the medical field, that psychic connection to their body will always exist, which creates the incredible potential to hone their body into whatever they wish.

This is a Pluto placement where we can see powerful athletes and/or those who find literal and figurative transformation and empowerment via the body. This can very much feel like a body-spirit connection, where one feeds the other.

PLUTO IN THE SEVENTH HOUSE

Along the Descendant, the Plutonian journey manifests through serious romantic relationships, similar to what we see with Venus-Pluto aspects. The process of growth and evolution plays out on the stage of committed partnerships, with each serious relationship offering up potent evolution in some way, for better or worse.

With Pluto in the house of close relationships, we can see both a fear of and a desire for the intimacy of deep one-on-one relationships. In fact, there may be a desire for a romantic relationship that feels very storybook and/or all-consuming. However, there is an equally strong resistance that can show up alongside that desire. That's because this placement can indicate a lot of pain and difficult experiences in love. We can see control, abuse, and loss. These are the people who have been through some pretty extreme situations when it comes to love, and over time a deep-seated mistrust and fear might have taken root. These individuals must also be careful not to project onto their partners and/or become controlling or abusive themselves.

However, with Pluto in the seventh house, we again are seeking to change the conversation and move from being transformed through the pain of love to being transformed through the soft, healing, and supportive qualities that a healthy relationship can offer. Those with a seventh house Pluto will be forced to circle back to close relationships and all they entail time and again, ideally finding a way to shed their fears, insecurities, and pain in favor of something more fulfilling and supportive. It is, after all, by allowing themselves to actually get close to people that real empowerment and transformation can begin.

Your Plutonian Superpower

With Pluto in the seventh house of committed relationships, your power lies in the way you love. Yes, the way you love is intense, but it is also transformative. Something about the type of love you offer to others truly rewires who they are, and your impact is long-lasting—maybe even lifelong. Seventh house lovers often experience exes who come back to them time and again, professing their love and/or sharing how the love they experienced from you was unlike anything else they've been able to find since. Similar to those with Pluto in the eighth house, you change those you love in profound ways.

PLUTO IN THE EIGHTH HOUSE

In the eighth house, the Plutonian journey is about transformation around sex, period, similar to what we see with Mars-Pluto aspects. Of the twelve houses in the chart, this is the one where Pluto might be considered to be at home, as almost all the themes of this house are the same as for the planet of the Underworld.

As with any point or planet contained within the eighth house, there is a lifelong journey of life, death, rebirth, and the transformation that comes along with it for those with Pluto here. In that sense, Pluto dials up the intensity of this journey even more. Here, the individual is grappling with themes of power, control, passion, and sex. What does it mean to be empowered when it comes to one's sexuality? That is the ultimate question.

In that sense, for those with Pluto in the eighth house, sex is a powerful avenue for transformation in life—likely through both enjoyable avenues and not-so-enjoyable ones. Again, the goal is to stop learning lessons through the pain of sexuality (such as shame or abuse) and instead learn through the healthy, enjoyable, and liberating qualities it can bring. Whatever that means is entirely subjective to the Plutonian person, but finding acceptance and joy around their sexual nature is key.

Outside of that, the question around shared resources within partnerships will also play a supporting role with Pluto in the eighth. It's true that these lovers may find themselves in relationships where money has often been unbalanced or possibly used as a means of control at some point. Finding a relationship where sharing and collaboration act as a source of support instead can also act as a catalyst for growth.

Your Plutonian Superpower

The cohesion between Pluto and the eighth house is unmatched, as the themes of this planet and this house are virtually one in the same. This makes Pluto in the eighth a particularly sexy, erotic placement.

Because of this, your superpower lies in your sexual energy, period. You possess a mysterious, alluring aura that is laced with the promise of sexual pleasure and fulfillment. There may be something about you that ignites the process of healing and transformation in others thanks to your ability to dive deep into the souls of other people. Your capacity for true intimacy—both emotionally and sexually—is your power. You change those you touch.

PLUTO IN THE NINTH HOUSE

With Pluto in the ninth house of religion, spirituality, and philosophy, we see an interesting journey around the idea of faith. The ninth house asks us about what we believe in that's higher or bigger than ourselves. In many ways, it is the house of the Divine, and with Pluto's influence here, there's something about religion and/or spirituality as a whole that makes these individuals ill at ease. Think religious trauma, for example. Perhaps they were raised in an extremely religious household. Maybe they were raised in a cult. Maybe they grew up in a totally atheist household. Again, the possibilities are endless, and with Pluto we are always looking to the extreme ends of the spectrum. No matter what the case may be, the beliefs of someone with this placement tend to be fundamentally at odds with those of their family and maybe even those around them to a greater extent. However, the spiritual path is an essential one for them, as is freedom in general.

Individuals with Pluto in the ninth house need the freedom to strike out into the world, to explore lands and cultures far and wide, and to greet as many different kinds of people and ways of existing as possible. Through firsthand experiences with different cultures and groups and seeing what they believe and how they live, the Pluto person is able to then turn around and develop their own philosophy and set of beliefs. This subjective set of morals and ethics and truths is the key to empowerment. Without it, these folks will flounder. And by allowing themselves to figure out their Truth (with a capital T!), the process of transformation can begin.

Your Plutonian Superpower

The ninth house is an especially spiritual position for Pluto in the chart. For those with this planet in the house of religion, spirituality, philosophy, and beliefs, there is a powerful, innate understanding of all things spiritual. These lovers have strong morals and ethics and can make profound teachers, able to guide others to higher truths.

Certainly we can see the potential for zealous religious leaders, philosophers, and spiritual teachers of all kinds with this placement. Because the ninth house also rules over academics, there is a path to power through higher education as well. These lovers could unearth novel information that significantly changes what we know about a subject, for example. There can also be strong connections to other cultures, languages, and lands.

PLUTO IN THE TENTH HOUSE

In the tenth house of our public-facing selves, Pluto is highly visible. More than with any other position of Pluto, the journey of transformation here lies within the career and finding one's purpose in life.

One of the main themes of Pluto in the tenth house manifests for these folks as struggling to know what they want to be when they grow up. There's something about working that is a source of great pain and disempowerment. Certainly we have to consider the question of money here, as that is a key component around the career. However, the wound really lies deeper than that. These individuals may struggle to find work or a direction that feels fulfilling, instead winding up in dead-end jobs or work situations that drain their life force. It's necessary for them to do some serious soul-searching around what kind of job would actually check their boxes, a tall order to be sure.

The other key component of Pluto in the tenth house surrounds the question of authority. At some point, these folks will probably find themselves in a job with an abusive boss. There is a journey around not allowing themselves to be taken advantage of by those in positions of authority, as well as learning how to have productive relationships with higher-ups that are rooted in respect—respect that goes both ways. The key to evolution here is finding their own inner authority and learning how to wield it in a way that makes *them* a good leader.

With Pluto in the opposite house from the fourth, there may also be issues in their relationship with their father, and a journey around healing that, too.

Your Plutonian Superpower

Without a doubt, the superpower of Pluto in the tenth house is one of authority, dominance, fame, and power. These Plutonian babes are incredibly capable leaders who possess the potential to accomplish a great deal when aligned with their true purpose or calling. They can gain a reputation for their passion, intensity, and drive and are magnetic, charismatic creatures. Once tapped into their Plutonian potential, they can act as catalysts for great change within their communities.

PLUTO IN THE ELEVENTH HOUSE

In the eleventh house, the Plutonian journey plays out through one's social circles and community. Whereas the seventh house focuses specifically on close, one-to-one relationships, the eleventh house is all relationships, with friends, family, lovers, neighbors, and coworkers. In a way, this placement is relationship karma on steroids.

Individuals with their Pluto in the eleventh house struggle to fit in perhaps more than anyone else. Certainly the concept of community feels foreign to them. They may struggle to maintain relationships or to connect with anyone who seems to be a good match. There may be issues of control within friendships or relationships in general that come forward and/or issues with betrayal. There is a lifelong journey around truly understanding what community means and hunting for their group.

It's very important that those with Pluto in the eleventh house are able to find people who truly see and understand them. It's likely that they feel they have to constantly translate their soul to others in order to really be seen or understood at all. They probably feel they're on the outside looking in on the rest of us and may not know why.

Being able to throw themselves into a social cause of some sort can help these individuals find the community they're looking for. Because we're looking at the eleventh house through the lens of Pluto, joining a group or cause that falls in line with Plutonian themes can be helpful for these lovers, too. Think kink, sex work, or working with those who are usually considered the outcasts of society in some way, such as people who are homeless or struggling with addiction. When those with this Pluto placement seek to empower their community, they in turn are able to empower themselves.

Your Plutonian Superpower

Lovers with Pluto in the eleventh house are the ultimate liberators of those around them. Because Pluto deals with taboos—and ultimately breaking them—those with this placement are able to bring people together who are normally on the outskirts of society in some way and help them find their community while breaking through stigmas. Because we have an extreme amount of power contained within our Pluto placement, these folks can do a lot for their community and help to build, create, and dismantle structures as needed. They are especially equipped for working with addicts, sex workers, etc.

PLUTO IN THE TWELFTH HOUSE

Pluto in the twelfth house is a rather interesting position for the Lord of the Underworld. In the last house of the natal chart, Pluto is locked away behind the veil of the subconscious and may not play as overt of a role as it does everywhere else in the chart. However, that doesn't mean Pluto is any less powerful here. On the contrary, because these lovers have to work extra hard to engage with the transformative power of Pluto, their issues around this planet may feel that much more pronounced.

Certainly the themes of dreams, mental health, and spirituality come forward here. Those with Pluto in the twelfth are likely to have very vivid dreams—maybe even downright prophetic ones. Anything they can do to dive deep into the themes of the subconscious and psychology, mysticism, and spirituality will unlock their journey to transformation and evolution.

Taking care of their mental health is of the utmost importance here, and taking the time to understand their own psyche can help exponentially.

It's important to remember that one of the themes assigned to the twelfth house is self-sabotage. Because we repress and bury things here, all our unhealthy coping mechanisms claw their way to the surface and come out sideways. Again, it's difficult to overstate the importance of self-awareness with this Pluto placement. A certain strength is required to take an honest look at ourselves and all the deep-seated issues we avoid, but that's exactly what Pluto asks for. Therapy (and the like) can be extremely helpful for these individuals and is something I strongly recommend.

Your Plutonian Superpower

With Pluto in the twelfth house, there is an extreme amount of psychic power. It's likely these lovers are vivid dreamers and have an innate, natural connection to the otherworldly. They are able to understand the subconscious motivations of others and to easily penetrate the surface and get into the depths of someone's soul. Because of this, they crave deep connections with others and can assist those around them in really unearthing the parts of themselves that they may not see or understand to help facilitate healing and growth.

These lovers would also do well helping those who are isolated in some way, such as working with those who are incarcerated, in hospitals, etc.

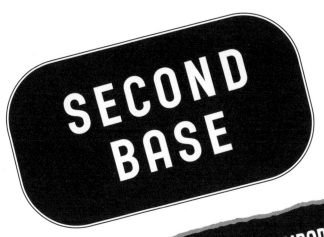

SECOND BASE

ASTEROIDS, ASPECTS, AND OTHER IMPORTANT POINTS

In this next section of the book, we depart entirely from the planets and move into a branch of astrology that is a bit more obscure and nuanced: the asteroids. In many ways, this is the cutting edge of astrology, as asteroids are only now beginning to be studied, understood, and integrated into popular astrological practices. For example, you may be familiar with Chiron, an asteroid that is often included when calculating a chart.

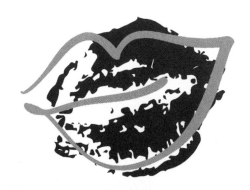

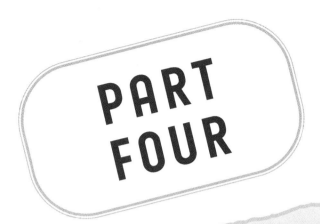

PART FOUR

ASTEROIDS AND IMPORTANT POINTS

Now, it's important to start off by saying there are thousands, maybe even tens of thousands, of asteroids to explore. It can quickly become overwhelming and, in my opinion, muddy up the chart. Most astrologers—myself included—tend to narrow our exploration down to just a handful of asteroids and other important points that have the most relevance and/or influence, which we will be exploring here.

Outside of asteroids, this section also includes the Vertex and the lunar nodes, which play an important role in fate and the evolutionary journey of the soul.

11
JUNO ⚵

In astrology, the asteroid Juno represents the archetype of the spouse. In many ways, Juno moves a step beyond the typical relationship dynamics that Mars and Venus point to and can tell us a lot about the type of committed partner we will be. It can also reveal the things we value in these committed partnerships and can speak more directly to the kind of loyalty we value within our long-term connections. In the chart, this asteroid represents our desire to enter into a lasting union, to build a future and a life with someone else. This is where we can see the characteristics we consider to be essential when entering into a bond with someone who is our equal.

The influence of Juno is strongest when in close connection with another planet or angle, such as on the Descendant (seventh house cusp), which also points to committed, intimate partnerships and marriage. However, even if Juno is by itself somewhere in the chart, the influence is still there. Juno also plays an important role in synastry when looking at compatibility between two (or more) people's charts. Here are some key characteristics of Juno through the signs.

JUNO IN ARIES

In Aries, Juno craves passion, adventure, and courage. There is an inherently fiery nature to this position that craves constant action, independence, and a certain amount of leadership or dominance.

JUNO IN TAURUS

The keyword for this placement is stability. Juno in Taurus desires an unwavering steadiness in their partner and relationship, as they, too, are steadfast. They crave safety, peace, predictability, and a level of financial abundance as well.

JUNO IN GEMINI

In Gemini, Juno hunts for open and honest communication. These are people who tend to get bored easily and are looking for someone smart, engaging, and fun. They value lightness, versatility, and fun.

JUNO IN CANCER

Juno in Cancer is deeply sensitive, nurturing, and family-oriented. Like with Juno in Taurus, safety is a key component for those with Juno in Cancer. They crave an ever-deepening connection and desire mutual caregiving.

JUNO IN LEO

There is a dramatic flair that is present in any Leo placement, and Juno in this sign is no exception. Juno in Leo desires a grand show of love and the need to feel special in their partner's life, as their partner is special in theirs. This Juno position in particular is fiercely loyal.

JUNO IN VIRGO

In Virgo, Juno is service-oriented, valuing acts of service as a love language, as well as communication. They want a quiet life and someone who is reliable and values health and cleanliness.

JUNO IN LIBRA

In many ways Juno is considered to be at home in Libra, the sign of partnership and equality. This position of Juno strives for harmony, balance, and fairness in their relationships, valuing an even give-and-take. Compromise is very important to those with Juno in Libra.

JUNO IN SCORPIO

Scorpio brings an intensity wherever it hangs out. For those with Juno in the scorpion's lair, a relationship that merges mind, body, and soul is the only acceptable connection. Emotional depth and sexual intimacy are key for these folks, and they are ready to embrace the ecstasy and agony of life with the right person.

JUNO IN SAGITTARIUS

Adventure and experience are the lifeblood of a relationship for Juno in Sagittarius. They want to do life with someone and will wither on the vine with someone who is more of a homebody. They have a certain zest for life and tend toward optimism, and it's important that their partner bring the same invigorating energy.

JUNO IN CAPRICORN

For Juno in Capricorn, the name of the game is commitment. These people are very clear about their long-term goals and values when it comes to partnerships, and they're looking for someone who is, too. They value integrity above all else and are looking to find someone who appreciates their wisdom and can also offer up their own.

JUNO IN AQUARIUS

Aquarius brings an air of unconventionality no matter where it hangs out in the chart. With Juno in the mix, these are folks who likely have some out-of-the-box ideas when it comes to partnerships. They are strong individuals who are looking for a strong partner who values freedom and originality. It is crucial that all partners involved accept and love each other for who they truly are.

JUNO IN PISCES

In Pisces, Juno is heartbreakingly romantic. These folks are looking to blur the boundaries between souls and enter into a soft, tender, and spiritually driven connection with someone else. Those with Juno in Pisces love to spend all their time together with their partner and value empathy, compassion, and unconditional love in its truest forms.

12
EROS ☄

As far as asteroids in sextrology are concerned, Eros is perhaps the most obvious and natural placement to consider. The word *eros* in Greek refers to physical, sexual love. It is the type of love that contains passion, lust, and desire. Everything that is physical, carnal, and insatiable is tied up in this asteroid. It embodies eroticism in a visceral, unbound way.

In the birth chart, Eros represents the way we express this physical passion. It can also show the level or extent of our eroticism. The sign it's in represents our desire, our hunger, the type of sex we crave on a cellular level. It shows what we find to be absolutely *irresistible*.

Eros is the desire we feel that bypasses our good sense and unlocks our primal desires. It's where we become obsessed, full to the brim with desire, and can become single-minded.

This asteroid describes our turn-ons, kinks, and sexual style. The sign it sits in may also point to the sign you are attracted to the most, as they naturally embody the sexual energy you crave. Eros mostly travels within the orbit of Mars, which might explain its deep links to mind-blowing sex.

As with all asteroids, the closer Eros is to another planet or angle in the chart, the greater its influence will be, in this case in terms of our sexual expression. Having Eros conjunct Venus, for example, increases the importance of sex in our romantic connections and may also boost the sex drive in general. Having Eros in a harsh square aspect to Saturn may dampen the sex drive, or it may feel very stop-and-go. Unlocking the nature of Eros in our chart is one of the more literal keys to being able to honor our sexual desires in a real way. Let's take a look at the characteristics of Eros through the signs.

EROS IN ARIES

An Aries Eros is someone who quickly becomes attracted and infatuated. Their instincts drive their sexual attraction and they tend to live in the heat of the moment, letting all else fall away as they pursue the object of their desire. As with all Aries placements, we see the quintessential intensity of passion with Eros in Aries. Initiating is never the issue; it is the follow-through that may not always be there. The flames of desire ignite quickly and can leave just as fast. Because of how fast these lovers burn through their emotions, they may come off as a bit erratic or fickle in their desires.

Again, this is where the heat of the moment becomes the focal point for Eros in Aries. Their full attention is rooted in the pursuit, which is really what gets them off. If there is some form of competition involved in the pursuit, even better. Aries is nothing short of dominant and loves an opportunity to show off just how dominant they can be.

Those with Eros in Aries aren't as giving or prone to deep emotions during sex as other placements, but they are full of passion while it lasts. In a way, Eros is at home in Aries, as this asteroid is about our embodiment of the physical expression of our passion, and everything about Mars-ruled Aries expresses itself physically.

Because of how quickly their desires spark and ignite, these lovers are also turned on by situations that get off the ground quickly. There's nothing an Aries Eros loves more than a potential lover who matches their energy and acts as the match to their kindling, ready to embrace the wildfire.

EROS IN TAURUS

In sensual Taurus, Eros takes on a much different shape. Unlike Eros in Aries, an Eros in Taurus does not enjoy competition when it comes to love. On the contrary, they could not be more turned off by it. These lovers can be jealous and deeply possessive of their partners and can be prone to wanting to "own" them in some way. Depending upon your personality, that quality can be more or less appealing.

In true Taurus fashion, this position of Eros speaks to a simple yet steadfast lover who gets off on long-term pursuits rather than the in-the-moment ones of Aries. A Taurus Eros is gluttonous in their sexual desires and can be very hands-on, preferring a full-body experience that activates all the senses. Remember that their earthy nature connects them to everything sensual. They want to feel, smell, see, and taste it.

Ultimately, thanks to their inherent Venusian energy, these people are happiest when in a committed partnership or at least with a steady, reliable sexual partner whom they trust. Safety is of the utmost importance to Eros in Taurus. They thrive on predictability, and in that sense they like to know what they can expect and will easily settle into something consistent once that trust has been established.

EROS IN GEMINI

With Eros in inquisitive and curious Gemini, we find individuals who are deeply interested in everything. These lovers prefer to be knowledgeable when it comes to sex, having spent plenty of time reading, researching, and experiencing as much variety as possible. These are the people who are prone to writing love letters and are most likely to be caught curled up in a corner reading smut. Thanks to Mercury (the ruler of Gemini), they are turned on by language, whether written or spoken, and they absolutely prefer erotic talk in the bedroom. In fact, their true pleasure may lie in the foreplay of dirty texts back and forth all day, building up the heat before getting together. Because of the insatiable curiosity of Eros in Gemini, this is also the position that points to the potential for voyeurism.

Just as with any other Gemini placement, it takes a lot to keep Gemini Eros lovers engaged and interested. Truly the biggest turn-on for them is intelligence. They value communication above all else, so someone who can speak on a variety of topics and is ready to talk to them about their relationship—sometimes endlessly—really gets their gears going.

EROS IN CANCER

In sensitive Cancer, Eros transforms into the picture of care and nurturing. The sexual connection will always need to be there along with the emotional one, as the two inevitably go hand in hand for these lovers. They seek out a deeply psychic and emotional transformation through sex, hoping for renewal through a meeting of the flesh. Depending on their current state of self-worth, they are prone to using sex as an escape or coping mechanism that may not exactly be healthy. These lovers are at their best when they feel good about themselves and can experience the deep spiritual connection in love and sex that they truly desire.

Thanks to their inherent intuitive gifts, these lovers possess the gift of knowing what their partners want and need in the bedroom. Similar to Eros in Taurus, those with a Cancer Eros need to establish a sense of safety and trust before they will open themselves up sexually. Once they do, however, their intuition makes them incredibly skilled lovers.

Because Cancer rules over the chest and stomach in astrology, those with Eros in the sign of the crab love a good set of tits—whatever that means to them. They may also enjoy a good-looking midsection, again according to their subjective preferences. This is also a position of Eros where we see dom-ination come into play, with Cancer often sliding into the role of the submis-sive. Despite being a cardinal sign, Cancers tend to be more doting and eager to please, usually falling into a position of being told what to do instead of the other way around. Depending on the other positions in the chart, however, the in-charge nature of this cardinal placement may come out every so often.

Similar to Eros in Taurus, possessiveness can be an issue with a Cancer Eros. These people often fall in love with their sexual partners and therefore may struggle to engage in anything casual.

EROS IN LEO

In Leo, Eros takes on a dramatic flair. There is nothing these lovers adore more than compliments and attention—true of any Leo placement. Flattery will get you everywhere with the cosmic lion, and they have a strong need to feel special. Leo loves to show off and be shown off. Keep in mind that they will show off their partners as well.

Eros in the sign of Leo is where we see a strong loyal streak. These individuals are more loyal than most and expect that loyalty to be shown in return. They're also incredibly passionate and tend to feel threatened or cagey if they see that passion waning. Remember that Leo is the sign that presides over sex, so especially with Eros here, we see a strong need to express that passion through sexual acts.

A Leo Eros is prone to autoerotic behavior, driven by their many fantasies. Similar to Eros in Pisces, those with a Leo Eros tend to have their head in the clouds, but their fantasies definitely surround sex and passion more so than straight-up love. Because of this, they are full of flirtation and infatuation. It's one way they try to keep the passion alive.

Beyond this, Eros in Leo gets off on the way they think their partners feel about them. These lovers are highly focused on the desire they believe others possess for them, whether it's rooted in reality or not. Remember, too, that Leo rules over the ego, and these lovers tend to have a lot of it (and a lot of pride) tied up in their connections.

EROS IN VIRGO

In analytical Virgo—which also represents the archetype of the Virgin—Eros manifests in a very curious way. These lovers are prone to overthinking when it comes to sex, a habit they may have to work hard to break free from. The flip side of this is that we see a deep attraction to intellectualism, a sexual intellectual if you will, where a meeting of the minds becomes both important and erotic. The analytical nature of Virgo also has these lovers thinking about sex from their partner's point of view, which creates a giving, sensitive nature as well as a bit of a voyeur, though it may be more self-voyeurism than anything else.

Because many Virgo placements struggle with their sexuality and general approach to sex, those with a Virgo Eros may go through phases of both celibacy and promiscuity as they waver back and forth on their journey to integrating their comfort around sex. Throughout this process they may struggle with being shy, if not a bit awkward. The part about Virgo that is perhaps a bit ironic is that they tend to actually be kinky and closeted freaks! Once they become comfortable with their desires and themselves, we see this side emerge more fully.

Outside of this, Eros in Virgo is highly concerned with health and the body. They may be quite picky, if not a bit neurotic, about the environment in which sex occurs and the people participating in it. Generally speaking, though, they have a healthy approach to sex, prioritizing health and safety above all, and they expect their partners to do the same.

EROS IN LIBRA

Just like any other Libra placement, Eros in Libra is incredibly charming. These lovers are flirtatious and know how to embody their own beauty, often catching the eye of plenty of potential suitors. In the bedroom, they are all about equality and an exchange of pleasure, at least in theory. In practice these lovers tend to be much more focused on their partners and can forget their own needs in favor of someone else's! In that sense, these people tend to get off on their partner getting off.

Naturally, a Libra Eros loves the idea of love and enjoys the social aspects of the game of cat and mouse we all play to some extent. This can be so true that once a relationship (or whatever kind of connection) settles into more of a routine, they get bored and jump ship—likely to hit up one of the many other admirers they have.

Outside of this, we see people who are attracted to all things aesthetically pleasing with Eros in Libra. These people love art, music, fashion, beauty, and so on.

EROS IN SCORPIO

We see an especially erotic position of Eros in the sign of Scorpio. In many ways, you might think of Eros as being at home in Scorpio. These lovers are intense and possess an insatiable appetite where sex and desire are concerned. They crave everything Eros promises, embodying all the natural qualities of this asteroid. As with all Scorpio placements, Eros in Scorpio lovers are intense, looking to understand their partners inside and out, forever on the hunt for an experience that merges mind, body, and soul.

A Scorpio Eros is fearless when it comes to love, sex, and intimacy, which is very similar to the vibes we see with a Scorpio Venus. Once someone has captured their attention, they become unflinchingly focused on them. They're extremely passionate and full of an almost animalistic desire and magnetism that others can easily sense, though they may not reveal these parts of themselves outright. There is very little these lovers aren't willing to do or try with a willing partner—the more intense (and kinky) the better!

As the other Mars-ruled sign (traditionally), Scorpio has a natural association with sex, and people with Eros here tend to spend a lot of time thinking about it and having it. Their sharp intuition gives them the ability to know how to get under people's skin in a way that has plenty of potential lovers heating up. Because of that intuition, a Scorpio Eros knows how to please.

EROS IN SAGITTARIUS

People with Eros in Sagittarius are quintessential sapiosexuals. They are smart and are turned on by people who are passionate about knowledge and hunger for new experiences. Certainly these lovers are *fun*. They love to laugh and crack jokes and often find witty banter to be an excellent lubricant to get the sexual energy flowing. They tend to see sex as a sport or a sparring event, at least in the beginning. In that sense, Eros in Sagittarius can enjoy the hunt or the game, similar to those with Eros in Aries.

As with all Sagittarius placements, Eros in Sagittarius takes a starkly open and honest approach to sex. These lovers will tell you exactly what they think about it, which may or may not be a bit shocking. They are always looking for new experiences when it comes to love and intimacy and need a partner who possesses that same sense of adventure. Keep in mind that they aren't the mushy type and are prone to fleeing the scene if a connection feels too restricting or overdone. Especially in Sagittarius, Eros may be looking for more of a fling than anything else.

These lovers in particular often have a thing for accents, as Sagittarius is connected to world travel and foreign cultures. They may connect with people from different backgrounds of all kinds, finding the variety to be erotic and stimulating.

EROS IN CAPRICORN

Lovers with a Capricorn Eros have an incredibly strong yet controlled libido. Their sex drive is high to be sure, and the earthy nature of Capricorn makes them very sensual, albeit a bit reserved.

Certainly these individuals like to be in control—it is Saturn that rules Capricorn, after all. We can see this sense of control manifest not only in their tendency to be dominant in bed but also in their strong self-control.

Like all other positions of Capricorn, Eros in Capricorn has a propensity toward privacy. They are not fans of PDA or grand gestures in public, so there's a need to get them alone before they are ready to open up, whether emotionally, sexually, or both. There is a grounded nature to these lovers that makes them powerful and focused—luckily for their partners, that focus is on them! The staying power of Saturn grants Eros in Capricorn incredible stamina and the ability to go and go and go again.

EROS IN AQUARIUS

Eros in Aquarius lovers are attracted to the unusual, quirky, and unexpected. It's hard to categorize the "type" they have, outside of it simply being strong individuals who are unique in some way. Those with Eros in Aquarius love variety, both in the types of lovers they have and in their sexual experiences—something new and weird is what excites them. This position of Eros is especially interesting because, as far as eroticism is concerned, Aquarius is the sign that tends to prefer the idea of sex more than the actual act. In that sense, these lovers may find eroticism in noncontact scenarios or find themselves feeling more desire when their person (or people) isn't physically around, preferring to sext or send photos and videos, for example. People who are aloof and detached often end up as the object of their desire as well.

Similar to Gemini and Virgo, Aquarius finds intellectualism and communication sexy. Aquarius is a curious, intelligent sign, and those with Eros here find people who can keep up with their widely varying interests and topics to be irresistible. They are also attracted to strong individuals who may not fit into a mold.

EROS IN PISCES

Eros in Pisces lovers are chameleon-like, shifting, changing, and adapting to the desires of their partners. Their ability to do this lies in the Piscean gift of being able to see the beauty in all types of people and understand their deepest desires. In the case of Eros in Pisces, this psychic gift manifests sexually and romantically.

While these lovers do have their own preferences in bed, they get off on being able to give their lovers what they want the most. Pisces is all about fantasy, after all, and there's nothing these individuals love more than embodying that fantasy for someone else.

More than any other position of Eros, though perhaps rivaled by Eros in Cancer, Eros in Pisces craves a deep emotional connection when it comes to sex. This isn't to say they can't have flings or casual sex, but Pisces, who blurs the boundaries of all things, seeks to connect heart, body, and soul and will have the most fulfilling connections where the emotional intimacy also exists.

Generally speaking, a Pisces Eros is attracted to sensitive, artistic types and those who are mystical, spiritual, and experimental with the boundaries of human expression.

13

VESTA ⚶

The final asteroid we'll look at in this book is Vesta. In astrology, Vesta represents the eternal hearth: the flame that burns without end. The asteroid's namesake is rooted in the Vestal Virgins of old, who spent their lives as priestesses devoted to the goddess Vesta, living in her temple and tending to the devotional hearth that they kept burning nonstop. In the birth chart, Vesta represents the commitment we have to ourselves (and the corresponding area of our lives) that exists within us naturally, outside of the influences of things like a job or other responsibilities that are thrust upon us. It is where our heart naturally lies, where we find joy and fulfillment by acting in service or devotion.

Personally, I adore this asteroid. I find Vesta to be a particularly poignant placement to explore, as it points beautifully both to where we show up for ourselves and whom and what our heart implicitly belongs to. It is the heart's most natural home.

As with any asteroid, Vesta plays a stronger role when it has a close connection to another planet or angle, but it's important to get to know regardless. Here are some key components of Vesta throughout the zodiac.

VESTA IN ARIES

This position of Vesta is truly devoted to embracing one's personal power, perhaps more so than any other possible placement. It is here that we see a devotion to passion, ambition, sexual prowess, and the self. It's important for individuals with Vesta in Aries to be able to embrace the more dominant and fiery qualities within. Though they may crave a connection, they are also quick to move on if the connection isn't serving them. These people have no issue being on their own.

VESTA IN TAURUS

Individuals with a natal Vesta in Taurus are devoted to pleasure and abundance above all else. This is a deeply sensual position that requires them to be able to fully embrace this part of themselves. It's important for them to be able to take things as slowly as they wish, relishing the various pleasures of the flesh, whether through food, fine clothes, or sex. In a relationship, it's crucial for them to be able to take things slowly as well. If the relationship isn't a source of comfort and groundedness, Vesta in Taurus will move into resentment—and likely move on.

VESTA IN GEMINI

In Gemini, Vesta is devoted to learning. These individuals like to keep things fresh, fun, and stimulating and have a wide variety of interests, both in hobbies and in people! Again we see communication as a key component here. Remember that Gemini is ultimately looking to connect with others—usually more on an intellectual plane than anything else.

VESTA IN CANCER

Those with Vesta in Cancer are devoted to nurturing their loved ones. They may be very family-oriented and naturally dedicated to them as well. Cancer thrives on deep emotional connections and is highly protective of their own sensitive nature. Safety is important to them above all else, and if there is a situation—or a person—that they don't feel they can trust with their more tender parts, they are quick to leave. Don't forget that Cancer is also fiercely protective, both of themselves and of those they care about.

VESTA IN LEO

With Vesta in flashy Leo, we see a natural devotion to creativity and self-expression. As with all Leo placements, Vesta in this sign displays a certain amount of magnanimity and an ability to lead. Those with a Leo Vesta feel empowered when they are helping their inner circle of loved ones in some way and are valued for their unique qualities and perspective. Being appreciated and—let's be real—admired is highly important to Vesta here. They are looking both to stand out *and* to be accepted.

VESTA IN VIRGO

In Virgo, Vesta highlights dedication to service, organization, and detail-oriented work. A Virgo Vesta excels in roles that require precision, efficiency, and problem-solving skills. This is another position in the chart where we see people who may trend toward acts of service as a way to show their affection. Certainly health is also something they value, both in themselves and in their partners.

VESTA IN LIBRA

In the sign of the scales, Vesta emphasizes dedication to relationships, harmony, beauty, and justice. These individuals may be committed to creating balanced and fair partnerships and working toward social equality, ideals that extend to their romantic relationships especially. A Libra Vesta requires their partners to share their same need for fairness, love, and beauty and expects an even give-and-take.

VESTA IN SCORPIO

With Vesta in Scorpio, the focus is on depth, transformation, and intimacy. Those with a Scorpio Vesta may dedicate themselves to uncovering hidden truths, healing, or supporting others through profound changes. They are devoted creatures, period, and strive to cultivate intense, passionate connections through intimacy. In that sense, they are just deeply devoted in general and value others who share their same level of passion.

VESTA IN SAGITTARIUS

Vesta in Sagittarius indicates dedication to exploration, learning, and personal growth. These lovers find fulfillment through expanding their horizons, traveling, or pursuing higher knowledge. Like any other Sagittarius placement, Vesta in Sagittarius individuals possess an incredible zest for life and are looking to experience as much as they can. They value others who share these same motivations and may also be inclined to more spiritual connections.

VESTA IN CAPRICORN

In Capricorn, Vesta highlights dedication to career, ambition, and responsibility. These people may be driven to achieve success and recognition in their chosen field through hard work and perseverance. This is also a placement that values integrity and commitment. In true Capricorn fashion, they may feel responsible toward their loved ones in some way and are willing to take on a great deal.

VESTA IN AQUARIUS

Vesta in Aquarius emphasizes dedication to humanitarian causes, innovation, and social progress. Those with Vesta in this sign are deeply committed to serving the greater good and making a positive impact on society. They may be social justice activists or interested in technology, science, or innovation. There is also an important focus on freedom, equality, and the dissemination of knowledge with this placement.

VESTA IN PISCES

With Vesta in Pisces, the focus is on spirituality, compassion, and creativity. These lovers may dedicate themselves to helping others, fostering empathy, and expressing their imagination and dreams through artistic pursuits. Indeed, these are people who greatly value the power of the imagination and expressing all the fantasies locked within their hearts. Just like any other Pisces placement, Vesta here is deeply empathetic and wants to shower everyone and everything with love.

14

THE LUNAR NODES
☋ ☊

We'll wrap up our journey through the erotic birth chart with the lunar nodes, also referred to as the nodes of fate or destiny.

The lunar nodes are directly tied to our karmic path in life. The South Node sheds light on our default setting: the way we most readily show up in life, in both good ways and more difficult ways. Understanding this aspect of ourselves can help explain why we are the way we are, the patterns we perpetuate in our relationships, what gifts we naturally bring to the table, and so on.

The North Node is the highest calling of our chart—it's the entire reason we're here. Whereas the South Node points to the parts of ourselves we've already mastered, the North Node points to the parts of ourselves and our lives that we are here to develop. Understanding this aspect of ourselves is crucial to empowerment as a whole and is inextricably linked to what we need across our relationships and experiences in order to find true fulfillment.

I have included the nodes because they are an integral part of the human experience and are key to finding the deep pleasure and fulfillment we seek the most. Before moving forward, I would like to highlight the fact that it's normal for the North Node to feel weird, scary, or intimidating because it's unfamiliar. The entire theory behind this node rests on the fact that we haven't spent any time getting to know that side of ourselves. However, the secret to the North Node is that when we *can* bring ourselves to do what it asks of us, life gets easier. Doors begin to open to us that have, up until that point, remained closed. Experiences that we've craved for a long time begin to show up in our lives, and therefore true fulfillment begins to weave its way in. When we bring ourselves to do the North Node thing, we find that not only do we survive, but things actually work out in our favor, and work out better than we expected them to. Just some food for thought.

ARIES AND LIBRA

No matter which sign each node sits in, Aries/Libra is the relationship axis. While this is true to a certain extent with any nodal pairing, relationships play a much more literal role here. Any and everybody with these nodes in their chart will spend their lives working out everything through their relationships. Regardless of the position of the nodes—whether it's the North Node in Aries or vice versa—the true call here is for balance in some way, whether through being more focused on themselves or on other people. Because it takes two (or more) to tango, other people often act as mirrors or catalysts in some way.

In my opinion, a big part of the journey here is for these individuals to identify what a healthy and balanced relationship is: What does it look like? Feel like? Act like? And where on the spectrum of give-and-take are their relationships currently falling? Keep in mind that as we grow, evolve, and change, so do our connections, and so does our definition of balance.

North Node in Aries, South Node in Libra

With the South Node in Libra and the North Node in Aries, we see people who struggle with codependency and autonomy. These lovers love love and feel their best when they are in a relationship. Indeed, their entire lives may feel focused on finding a partner, and quite frankly they don't know how to be alone. In my experience, these are people who are serial monogamists. They are pretty much always in a serious relationship and flounder when they are forced to be single. Even when they are freshly out of a partnership, their focus immediately moves to finding the next person.

Are these individuals who know how to show up and be there for other people? Absolutely. The trouble comes when they give and give and give and prioritize everyone else's wants and needs over their own. In that sense, they are self-sacrificing and often lack the courage to stand up for themselves, which is where the North Node comes in.

As I've mentioned several times earlier in this book, Aries is the sign of the self and Libra the sign of the other. With Aries as the focal point of the North Node, there is a journey for these individuals around independence, standing up for themselves, and learning how to stand on their own two feet. To be honest, being single—and being happy about it—is a crucial piece of the puzzle for them. Now, does this mean they're doomed to be alone for the rest of their lives? Certainly not. They might, if they *choose* it, but it isn't a requirement. What *is* a requirement, however, is learning to prioritize themselves and what they want and need in relationships and life in general. There are lots of lessons around learning to value themselves and their desires as much as everyone else's. Remember that the ruler of an Aries North Node is Mars! Finding the courage to speak up and name what they want and need will set them free.

On the sextrology front, Mars is the planet of sex, so certainly there is an ask here around sex, physical expression, and passion. Moving the body and empowering the vitality within is the name of the game. Learning to be a bit more selfish in the bedroom is actually a good thing, as is focusing more on their own pleasure. I promise these lovers are givers in the bedroom with that South Node in Libra, and learning to assert themselves sexually will liberate them. Masturbating is a great thing for them, too.

South Node in Aries, North Node in Libra

With the South Node in Aries and the North Node in Libra, the focus is on relationships, period.

The South Node in Aries speaks to an interesting dichotomy. These are people who know exactly who they are. Indeed, they are passionate, driven, and highly focused on their desires. However, they also often experience a great deal of conflict within their connections. In my experience, these individuals have spent most of their lives feeling like they have to fight to get others to accept them, and/or they've been given the message that who they are isn't really a good thing. There's something about them just being themselves that seems to set people off or not sit well with others, which leaves them constantly experiencing conflict and turmoil with others.

The hard part about this, which is entirely subjective, is where the self-ishness of Aries comes in. Because we are always looking at the shadowy or unevolved characteristics of a sign with the South Node, it is a possibility that these individuals are selfish! Now, they may not see that as a problem—which, ironically, may be part of the problem. This is where real life comes in, and there are too many possibilities to dive into around the dynamics and circumstances they may have been forced to grow up in and so on. Regardless, there is an undeniable pull toward having to consider other points of view.

That's because the North Node in Libra points to a focus on other people. Certainly there are lots of lessons around compromise; very often these individuals have to learn the value of taking other people's wants and needs into consideration and learning to value their loved ones' desires just as much as their own. More than with any other nodal combination, relationships are the stage on which all their lessons will play out. I want to emphasize that the idea is to find *peace* within their relationships, to finally be able to put down their sword and exist in harmony, tranquility, and real, healthy love. Part of this means finding people who do love and accept them for who they are, while also learning how to show up and give—balance, in true Libra fashion.

On the sex front, we're looking to find an even give-and-take in the bedroom, likely with an emphasis on giving. Again, there's a need for these individuals to value their partner's pleasure as much as their own. Venus, the ruler of a Libra North Node, is all about pleasure, and in the temple of Libra everyone needs to give as well as receive. In that sense, the natural dominance that courses through the veins of an Aries South Node could benefit from giving up a bit of that power and control in favor of a bit more—dare I say it?—submission.

TAURUS AND SCORPIO

This Taurus/Scorpio position of the nodes is somewhat complex. Certainly relationships continue to be a big focus with this pairing, but the focus shifts from just relationships in general to trust, intimacy, pleasure, and resources. This nodal pairing folds in the question of sex more than any of the others, including Aries/Libra. While both sets of signs share the Venus and Mars rulerships, Taurus and Scorpio grapple with sensuality versus sexuality, respectively. Trust is also a central theme here, which is ultimately the underlying force behind all the surrounding questions with this nodal combination. Without trust, we cannot experience intimacy, we cannot foster a sense of stability or pleasure, we cannot embrace change, and we cannot come together and share ourselves and our resources in an effective, long-lasting way. More than with any other pairing of signs, trust is at the forefront of the nodal journey for Taurus/Scorpio.

North Node in Taurus, South Node in Scorpio

With the South Node in Scorpio and the North Node in Taurus, the journey is ultimately to move toward stability. In my experience, those with the South Node in Scorpio tend to come from a place of instability one way or another. These lovers have gone through some seriously intense hardships in their lives and know the journey of transmuting their pain into power all too well. They may feel they are relentlessly going through the death experience and having to endure experiences that change who they are entirely again and again and again.

The hard part about this nodal combination is that there's a fundamental part of these creatures that lives for the intensity. Certainly they possess the burning passion that Scorpio is known for, regardless of how the rest of their chart may work, and therefore they have to reconcile the parts of themselves that thrive in the intensity of their experiences, regardless of how painful they may be.

Whenever I explain to these individuals that their North Node in Taurus is asking for stability and to ultimately break free from the cycle of death and rebirth to find stability and peace, they tend to recoil, often feeling that the call of their North Node is rather boring. As someone whose chart is ruled by Scorpio, I do understand this. However, the call here is really for these individuals to find a way to turn the flames of passion into the fire that keeps them warm, offers light, and cooks their food, rather than the funeral pyre they're used to.

As far as sex is concerned, again we see the high sex drive and animal magnetism that Scorpio is known for. The North Node in Taurus isn't an ask to deny these parts of themselves, but rather to embrace the slow, sensual nature of Taurus. Indeed, slowing down in general is a key component of this nodal combination. In this case, sex may be somewhat weaponized—a common trait of Scorpio—and the North Node is asking them to invite in true pleasure and the true intimacy that can only be cultivated slowly, over time.

South Node in Taurus, North Node in Scorpio

With the South Node in Taurus, we see someone who downright resists change. As a reminder, Taurus thrives on stability, yes, but especially through the lens of the South Node, it's truly about *predictability*. Taurus works hard to establish a lifestyle that is constant, because it's what feels safest to them, which ends up manifesting as them wanting to know exactly what's going to happen all the time, and it being the same thing over and over and over. Pair that with the downright stubbornness of Taurus? Forget about it.

Because it's necessary to look at the South Node through a somewhat pessimistic lens, we see a fear of change here. The slow-moving nature of Taurus can turn into a timeless resistance that scarcely evolves at all, which is where the North Node in Scorpio comes in.

As the sign of transformation, Scorpio calls for these lovers to embrace the natural cycles of life, death, and rebirth that life demands. Nothing changes if nothing changes, and these individuals are here to shed the chains of complacency and stagnation. Through allowing their intuition and passions to come forward and guide them through life, they are able to learn that change can be a *good* thing, even if the unknown feels scary at first. In fact, the unknown can be downright exciting if you let it.

There is also a need to move toward greater depth in relationships. One of the hallmarks of the South Node in Taurus is having vapid, surface-level connections with others. These lovers may have plenty of acquaintances and casual friends, but it's unlikely they have ever really let someone in. Scorpio craves a merging of souls, a relationship that is all-consuming, mind, heart, body, and soul. Remember that Scorpio is fearless when it comes to intimacy, and they won't settle for anything less. This lifetime is about welcoming in these types of connections, cultivating depth and true intimacy, learning how to share resources with their serious partners, and following their passions and obsessions.

When thinking about the North Node in Scorpio in terms of sex, there is an obvious call for these individuals to embrace their sexuality. As I've mentioned a couple of times already, Scorpio rules over the genitals. Because this sign's traditional ruler is Mars, the planet of sex, there is a journey for these lovers around embracing the passion, the physical, the erotic. There is a need to take action around these things instead of waiting around passively or moving at a glacial pace, as Taurus tends to do. Following the fire within opens the doors to empowering the animal within.

GEMINI AND SAGITTARIUS

In Gemini and Sagittarius, the nodes have a much more lighthearted disposition than in Taurus and Scorpio. That doesn't mean the journey is any less difficult for people with this pairing, however. The nodal journey is difficult for everyone, regardless of the signs the nodes sit in.

In the case of Gemini and Sagittarius, we see a huge focus on communication, the small picture versus the big picture, learning, and beliefs. This is the first combo of the nodes that isn't so overtly about romantic and sexual relationships but focuses on more cerebral issues. That doesn't mean these lovers are free of relationship karma, however! It's just playing out on a different level than what we've covered thus far. Keep in mind that Gemini is the sign of the twins and therefore represents the self versus the other in a lot of ways, too. Plus, communication is one of the biggest components of any kind of connection.

North Node in Gemini, South Node in Sagittarius
Those with their South Node in Sagittarius are optimistic and funny and have an incredible faith in the Divine. This is thanks to their ruler, Jupiter,

who grants them such qualities. Because Sagittarius is a fire sign, through the lens of the South Node there is an inherent selfishness. While this isn't necessarily a bad thing, these lovers are known for being hyper independent, almost to a fault, if we're being honest. Especially with the South Node in Sagittarius, we see individuals who are sure about what they want and what they believe in, and they don't really care about or have time for anybody who would weigh them down. The big picture of their lives is clear, and you can either come along for the ride or not. Either way, they're going to do what they want to do.

Alternatively, the North Node in Gemini is all about the details. As optimistic and sure as these babes can be about what they want out of life, they aren't that great at figuring out the actual steps that have to be taken to make the big picture come together. The Gemini North Node is about learning how to zoom in on the minutiae and figuring out the step-by-step processes, the little things that come together to make up the whole. It's also about embracing and cultivating the curiosity to find interest in numerous different things instead of staying tied to one big ideal.

Inevitably for those with the North Node in Gemini, there is also a focus on communication and learning how to connect with other people. With Gemini, the sign of the twins, we are looking at the self versus the other and balance in relationships. Learning how to put themselves in other people's shoes, have an even give-and-take in conversations, and embrace other ways of looking at things is key. Because Gemini is an air sign, there's also a focus on practicality over the intuitive, faith-based approach of Sag.

Truly this nodal journey is about balance. The South Node in Sagittarius weighs too heavily on one side of the scale, and the North Node in Gemini is here to put a focus on the other, neglected side, which enables these lovers to find equilibrium in all things.

These same ideals show their face in the sexual journey of the North Node in Gemini. Embracing new ways of approaching relationships, sex, and love is key. For those with a Gemini North Node, learning to find opportunity and staying curious about alternative types of relationships and sexual expression will open the doors to evolution. In that sense, because there is such a focus on other people, learning to give in the bedroom, and finding value in that, is crucial. There may be a need for these individuals to really break down their philosophy on the erotic side of life and begin to question why they believe what they do, which can lead to greater self-awareness and understanding. Doing this through conversation with others can be mighty, mighty helpful.

South Node in Gemini, North Node in Sagittarius

When the South Node is in Gemini, we see someone who is chatty as hell. Thanks to Gemini being ruled by Mercury, the South Node in this sign grants these lovers the gift of gab and a busy, busy mind. On the one hand, these lovers are full of ideas and are highly adaptable and curious creatures. They are excellent at putting themselves in other people's shoes and appreciating the subjective experiences and perspectives that life brings along. They're likely very busy people who may seem to be constantly on the go. The downside to this placement, however, can have these people lost in the sauce by way of information overload, and with so many potential paths and interests they may have trouble committing to or truly following through on anything. Because Gemini is a highly relational sign, they may also spend too much time caught up in the obligations of their relationships, which is where the North Node comes in.

Ultimately, the North Node in Sagittarius is a call for greater independence and freedom. By nature, Sagittarians are hyper independent. As a fire sign, they display a certain self-centeredness that has them focusing on their own goals and desires. Now, let's not assign the negative connotations of self-centeredness here. On the contrary, leaning into more of what these lovers desire is actually what's best for them. They've spent too long being focused on others, and the duality that Gemini asks for is achieved through channeling all (or at least more of) that energy back into themselves. Part of doing this is achieved through embracing the big-picture perspective that Sagittarius rules over.

The call of the North Node in Sagittarius is truly to zoom out, to take on a higher vantage point that enables these individuals to see the big picture and therefore see how the details need to weave together to achieve that higher goal. In that sense, there's a call to commit to something, anything, and follow through.

When it comes to sex, I think the best way to understand the North Node in Sagittarius is to stop overthinking. Lovers with their South Node in Gemini will analyze everything to death, which can really kill the mood. For those with a Sagittarius North Node, learning how to get out of their head and into the moment makes way for more fun, excitement, and adventure to come through in general but especially in the bedroom. Sagittarius is here for the adventure and isn't concerned with all the what-ifs that may or may never come to fruition. For people with the North Node here, embracing this philosophy when it comes to hooking up will be liberating as fuck. The key to evolving their erotic self is opening themselves up to new people and new experiences and allowing the fire to fuel their desires.

CANCER AND CAPRICORN

With the nodes in Cancer and Capricorn, we shift from communication and learning to the axis of nurturing and the way a person's approach to this concept is expressed, through either emotional nurturing or more practical means, such as paying the bills. More than with any other nodal combo, family and career play a key role with Cancer/Capricorn, as do the themes of stability, authority, and safety. Certainly there is a question around the need for independence versus close relationships and trying to strike a balance between both, as one of these areas of life is too strong and is a detriment to the individual.

Beyond this, there is a question around the intuition, emotional connections, and the need for practicality.

North Node in Cancer, South Node in Capricorn

A person with the South Node in Capricorn is the quintessential workaholic. Similar to what we see with the South Node in Sagittarius, lovers with a Capricorn South Node are independent to a fault. That's due to the fact that they've had to take on responsibility from a very young age. There are plenty of different circumstances that could be the cause of this, but one way or another, the environment they grew up in required them to grow up quickly and learn how to take care of themselves and probably those around them. These are the kids who were told they were super mature for their age, or an old soul, or whatever. They're naturally very mature and indeed may seem to possess wisdom beyond their years, as is the true Capricorn way.

As grounded, wise, and realistic as those with the South Node in Capricorn may be, the chains of responsibility are heavy. There is a tendency to feel a need to be in control, to take their responsibilities *too* seriously, and to be rigid and fearful of being dependent on others. Yes, these individuals are driven, ambitious, and capable, but the sad reality is they're not used to getting their emotional needs met, which is where the North Node comes in.

Cancer is all about nurturing, especially on an emotional level. As Cancer is the sign that rules over the home, family, and foundations, the journey for individuals with the North Node here is all about finding that home base and place of love and safety that they've been craving all their lives. This is both an internal and an external journey. They must learn to prioritize and value the softer side of life, as connecting on a deeper emotional level and getting their emotional needs met is the missing piece of their lives that will bring them *true* fulfillment. Life isn't just about work and goals and ambitions and blah, blah, blah. These lovers are actually here to stop investing so much in their careers and instead focus on their close, important relationships. Note that one potential manifestation of a Cancer North Node is literally building a family and becoming a parent.

The sexual journey of this nodal pairing focuses on cultivating emotional intimacy and combining it with the physical. Sex becomes less transactional and evolves into something profound and beautiful when the emotional piece coexists with the sexual desire. This is all about embracing the softer, more tender side of sex. It's about lovemaking over fucking, period.

South Node in Cancer, North Node in Capricorn

When the South Node is in Cancer, we see individuals who hate having to be an adult. Oftentimes they feel painfully nostalgic for their adolescence, a time when they didn't have any responsibilities and they felt more carefree. Because of this, we see individuals who have a tendency to fall back on the support of other people, often their families, when the going gets tough. While there is an undeniable amount of support here, the problem comes when that support is too enabling and stifles their ability to grow and learn.

The call of the North Node in Capricorn, then, is for these people to become fully self-sufficient, to be able to take care of themselves on their own, no longer requiring the support of their loved ones in order to survive. It's about really taking it there with their dreams and ambitions.

While there is a great amount of emotional awareness and maturity with the South Node in Cancer, true fulfillment for these lovers isn't going to come through their close relationships anymore. Instead, it will only come through achieving their goals, through the payoff that comes with hard work and ambition and any accompanying recognition in the career. At some point in their journey, these lovers will realize how continuing to cling to the comforts of their youth is holding them back. Ideally this epiphany will spur them to move out and get their own place and, quite frankly, never look back. Of course family will always be important to these babes, but it's only when they start taking care of themselves and have the independence that comes from physically distancing themselves from their family that they can start living their lives the way they need to in order to grow and evolve.

The sexual journey of those with the North Node in Capricorn is about finding their inner authority and embracing and embodying it. No longer is it about submission or needing to wait until they are in love with someone. Instead, it's about finding their erotic power and taking control. Having the sex life they desire is key here. Obviously this could look any number of ways, but it's less about what it looks like and more about feeling rooted in their erotic energy. There is a commitment to embodying that power that the North Node in Capricorn demands. Playing a more active or dominant role in their sexual connections is also key. Capricorn is *in charge*, and these lovers are meant to be too.

LEO AND AQUARIUS

The nodal axis of Leo and Aquarius is a curious one. Certainly both signs point to a question of individuality and creative self-expression, but we also have to confront the question of the role of the individual versus the group. No matter which position each node is in, authentic self-expression is key here. However, depending on where the North Node lies, the focus is on either breaking away from the group or finding the group we fit into. There are moments for us to shine and moments for us to blend in, but no matter which moment we're in, we still have to be ourselves. There is an inevitable moment of having to grapple with the ego as well. Contrary to a lot of messaging in the spiritual community, we actually need our ego. We aren't here to eradicate it—and we couldn't even if we tried—but we are here to try and have the most awareness and healthy expression of it as possible. Such is the journey of this nodal axis. How can we use our individuality and gifts to serve ourselves and the group? Where have we sacrificed our true expression for the will of the masses and vice versa?

North Node in Leo, South Node in Aquarius

One of the beautiful things about people with the South Node in Aquarius is they're focused on community, social justice, and equality for all. They are often fantastic members of their community and are driven to support those around them. They're also probably quirky and full of idiosyncrasies—remember that Aquarius is a bit odd.

The trouble for these lovers comes when they lose themselves in the crowd and sacrifice who they really are for the group. Aquarians want to be themselves, to be sure, but they prefer to blend into the crowd rather than stand out. Those with Aquarius placements in general can struggle with feelings of alienation and being too different from those around them, preferring to hide within the confines of a group so their peculiarities go unnoticed. This is especially true for those with their South Node in Aquarius. However, the North Node in Leo will not stand for this.

The very nature of Leo *is* to stand out from the crowd. The Sun presides over Leo, which is all about the ego, illuminating the North Node path toward shining in everything that makes these lovers who they are. They are meant to shine in their uniqueness, channeling all their special qualities in a way that draws attention to them instead of hiding within the masses. And, yes, this is probably quite uncomfortable for them, but it's important to remember that we get rewarded in life through doing the North Node thing.

With the North Node in Leo, there is also a call around embracing their passions, similar to what we see with the North Node in Scorpio and Aries. The South Node in Aquarius is detrimentally detached, preferring to stay aloof and objective and free of emotion. Leo is the exact opposite. Thanks to their fiery nature, Leo feels everything, and they feel it strongly. Learning to be bold and passionate and creative, to allow the heart to come forward and take the steering wheel, will help these lovers evolve in the ways they truly crave. For those with a Leo North Node, life is about having the experiences they want to have and learning how to play, have fun, and live in the moment. One way to think about it is that it's not that deep. Sometimes doing things just because they're fun, because we want to, because it brings us joy, is more than a good enough reason. Remember that we're moving here from the cold and distant tundra of Saturn (ruler of Capricorn) to the warm, life-giving heat of the Sun (which rules Leo). Life is meant to be enjoyed, and that's what these babes are here to learn.

In that same vein, those with a Leo North Node are also here to apply those principles to sex! As I've mentioned plenty of times in this book, Leo is the sign that rules over sex. So more than for any other position of the North Node—yes, even North Node in Scorpio—the Leo North Node journey is about embodying their sexuality and being bold as fuck about it. No longer can these lovers remain detached in their relationships. They are here to embrace warmth and generosity and ardor, to allow their heart and passions to ignite the spark of life in them and to experience sex in all its wonderful glory. For those with the North Node in Leo, passion *must* be channeled physically, and entwining it with actual feelings is crucial. Being cool is out and being insanely full of life is in.

South Node in Leo, North Node in Aquarius

The South Node in Leo is a rather curious placement to have. While these lovers are warm, generous, and charismatic, possessing an innate popularity and magnetism, the question around identity and authenticity is a tricky one. The ruler of the South Node in Leo is the Sun, the very representation of who we are in astrology. Because of this, the karma these individuals are working out in this lifetime is actually *themselves*. As Leo is the only sign that is ruled by the Sun, these folks are grappling with karma in a way that nobody else is, which feels so very inherently Leo.

While you can bank on lovers with a Leo South Node being strong individuals, there's something about the circumstances they find themselves in time and again that is in direct conflict with them being able to show up as themselves. Indeed, it's likely they have been forced to play some kind of role, to wear a mask, for the approval and entertainment of other people. They may feel they're only accepted by others when they're playing the role of the court jester in some way. One thing I've read plenty of times in my journey as an astrologer is that people with their South Node in Leo were likely royalty in a past life or were at least well-to-do, and while that may be true for some of them, with the North Node in Aquarius that isn't the case anymore. On the contrary, these individuals probably had a difficult childhood in some way that crippled their ability to experience fun and joy and play. A truly strange dichotomy exists with the South Node in Leo, then, where we see the fiery nature of Leo imbue these lovers with passion and confidence and many unique talents, yet they aren't able to truly know or express themselves in an authentic way. Cue the North Node in Aquarius.

The Aquarius North Node asks these lovers to find a sense of community, it's true. Ultimately they are looking for the group of people they belong to, who see and love them just as they are, cultivating the environment they need to just be themselves for once. There may be a journey around learning to share and to place their identity within the correct group setting rather than stand alone. However, the need for individuality will always be present along this axis. Remember that despite the humanity-oriented focus of Aquarius, the reality of this sign involves a certain amount of distance or detachment. Yes, they want to share their vision and disseminate their knowledge, but they also want to be left alone to do their own thing. Thus the call is to find a correct balance of both: the individual versus the group, passion versus detachment, and, above all else, authenticity. Perhaps the best way to think about it is as a need to break free from the expectations of others and no longer be put in a box.

More than any other position of the South Node in astrology and sextrology, Leo brings forward the question of sex as a key issue. Leos are super sexual by nature, and because love and sex are difficult for them to separate, lovers with the South Node here have to grapple with using sex as a way to experience validation in their relationships. This is a somewhat curious journey, as Aquarius is so detached and aloof and often likes the idea of sex more than the actual act. This doesn't mean the call is for individuals with the North Node in Aquarius to stop having sex, but there is a big lesson around how their passions have led them astray, and learning to detach and approach things more objectively can help them have a healthier relationship with their sexual side and with love and romance in general. Yes, this might mean having less sex. But ultimately it means learning to approach sex in a way that is more authentic instead of using it as a tool for validation.

VIRGO AND PISCES

In this final pairing of the lunar nodes, we approach the idea of service. Something interesting to note about this duo is the fact that, in some branches of astrology, the South Node is considered to be in domicile, or at home, in Virgo, and therefore at home when the North Node is in Pisces. Whether this theory resonates with you or not is entirely subjective, but in my opinion it can be helpful to explore. What sort of implications exist for a person when their nodes are at home? Or the reverse?

I'll be honest: The Virgo/Pisces nodal combination can be a difficult one to have, and in my experience with others, they tend to agree. There are several reasons for this, which we will go over shortly, but at the heart of it all lies the theme of service, which inevitably brings forward the question of sacrifice. Acting in service to others is a hard thing to do precisely *because* it requires selflessness and sacrifice on our end. It's not something a lot of people necessarily want to do or would choose to do, but it is the ultimate act of love and is a beautiful thing to offer up to others. And in this case, it is also unavoidable.

Personally, I find this nodal journey to be reserved for the most evolved. I think it's the pinnacle of what it means to be human to truly walk the path of unconditional love. However, I do recognize that this path is not an easy one. If this happens to be your nodal combo, don't fret. Remember that life gets easier and more fulfilling when we embrace the call of our North Node.

North Node in Virgo, South Node in Pisces

Similar to the nodes in Gemini and Sagittarius, we again see the rulers of the nodes in Virgo and Pisces as Mercury and Jupiter (traditionally), respectively. We are grappling here with moving through both the spiritual and the mundane. In the case of the South Node in Pisces and the North Node in Virgo, these individuals are moving from the spiritual back into their mundane, everyday lives.

Now, I don't want "mundane" to equate to "boring" here. Those with their South Node in Pisces are inherently spiritual people, but as we are also dealing with the shadier side of Pisces, they are also people who tend not to live in reality. They may prefer solitude and isolation, which is fine, until it bleeds over into being downright avoidant, which is the hallmark of a Pisces South Node.

The flip side of this is a powerful and vivid imagination. Those with their South Node in Pisces are incredibly creative and empathetic and live in a beautiful dreamscape. Certainly there are plenty of gifts to channel here. But the tendency to live in the fantasy world of their heads and not tend to the responsibilities of their actual lives is all too real.

The North Node in Virgo is a call for these individuals to play a more active role in their lives—to get more involved and learn how to show the fuck up. There is a huge focus here on needing structure, routine, and organization and living more within their body. As boring or difficult as that may sound to them, learning how to be present and do the tasks that being an adult requires is absolutely crucial. Paying attention to their physical health is important as well.

This same idea extends to sex as well. For those with the South Node in Pisces, there is a tendency both to isolate from others and to use sex and relationships as a means of escape. While these lovers can certainly be romantic and idealistic, they may struggle to see their partners and/or the nature of their relationships for what and who they truly are. Because we have to look at the South Node through a somewhat negative lens, this is where the codependency of Pisces can show up. The call for a Virgo North Node, therefore, is to have better boundaries around all things erotic. Boundaries enable us to maintain clarity and be grounded in reality—an all-too-crucial part of evolution for these lovers. Learning to prioritize their health in all facets of love and sex will lead to evolution and open the doors to more fulfilling experiences.

South Node in Virgo, North Node in Pisces

With the South Node in Virgo and the North Node in Pisces, we see the complete opposite come forward. These individuals are moving from the tangible to the intangible, from a rigid routine and way of being toward a more fluid, spiritual life. Indeed, outside of maybe the North Node in Sagittarius, this is the most fundamentally spiritual journey of all the possible nodal combinations.

I'll be honest and say that in my experiences with people who have these nodes, the journey can feel quite difficult for them. There often comes a point in their lives when they are forced to grapple with having been highly successful, organized, and capable to now struggling to do much of anything. One example is struggling to maintain a routine or show up on time.

Now, this doesn't mean that those with the North Node in Pisces are doomed to a life of chaos or being unsuccessful. However, an unavoidable piece of this journey is to learn how to go with the flow, to embrace the unknown through a process of trusting the Divine and therefore trusting the unfolding of their path. So much of learning how to do that means letting go of control, which Virgo loves to have. It's also worth noting that a big lesson here is learning that there are many different ways of doing things and living one's life, and none of them are "right" or "wrong," which is a concept Virgo struggles with.

Beyond this, there is a call for self-compassion and forgiveness here. Those with their South Node in Virgo have a horribly mean inner critic and succumb all too easily to the trap of perfectionism. Learning to accept the reality that "perfect" does not exist, and therefore *they* will never be perfect but are still good enough just the way they are, will set them free.

Undeniably, for those with a Pisces North Node, there is also a journey around learning to listen to their intuition, to value the emotional side of life, and to embrace the softer, more creative side of themselves. Empathy, compassion, and idealism are the areas that need the most development here, and opening themselves up to connecting on deeper emotional and spiritual levels will become a stronger and stronger theme throughout their lifetime.

As far as sex is concerned, these lovers may have some self-consciousness around their sexuality, as is the Virgo way. Learning to accept this side of themselves and to foster deep love and tenderness around their erotic side is the call of the North Node in Pisces. Because Pisces is so very romantic, something about having more inherently romantic experiences can teach these lovers how to let go of the more transactional or rigid approach they normally have. They must learn to see the beauty in all things, including themselves, and to open themselves up to love, nurturing, and acceptance.

15
THE VERTEX Vx

In the birth chart, the Vertex isn't a planet or asteroid at all, but a physical point that exists at the intersection of the ecliptic (the path the Sun travels) and the prime vertical, which divides the ecliptic from front to back. Thanks to this intersection, the Vertex (often appearing as "Vx" in the chart) is always located in the right half of the birth chart, often falling in relationship-heavy houses such as the fifth, seventh, or eighth—though not always. It's important to note that in astrology, the right half of the chart is considered to be more relationship-focused anyway.

So why care about this imaginary point? Because the Vertex represents fate in our connections with other people.

This point in the chart is unlike anything else because it signals events, connections, and happenings that are outside of our control. Vertex-related occurrences manifest through no will or volition of our own, and in that sense they point to the people, places, and activities that we may attract into our lives without even being aware of it.

Now, it's important to understand that the energy of the Vertex isn't always active—we need something to awaken its energy. One of the ways this can happen is through a natal or transiting planet making some kind of aspect to our Vertex. However, what I have seen happen more often—and, I would argue, more powerfully—is coming into contact with someone who happens to have a planet or angle (such as their Ascendant) that is conjunct (right on top of) your own Vertex. For example, say you have your Vertex in Gemini and you meet someone who has their Sun in Gemini (or their Moon, or Venus, or Mars) at the exact same degree as your Vertex, and it suddenly turns into a life-changing whirlwind romance. Or maybe they become an important business partner, or the two of you get married, or they become a lifelong friend. You get the idea.

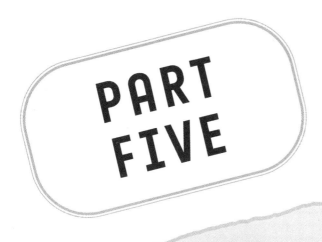

PART FIVE

ASPECTS

When we think about placements in relation to one another in sextrology, it colors the way these cosmic bodies interact with each other and the way we embody them. In a sense, because of these interactions, their influence becomes much stronger and they play a more important role in love, sex, romance.

16
THE ASPECTS

In my experience, aspects in the chart are one of the most confusing and difficult things for people to understand. That's okay—I would argue they're one of the more advanced pieces of the chart. However, they're also very important.

When we talk about aspects between planets, it means that the planets are positioned in such a way that they're speaking to each other. This link between two (or more) points in the chart becomes an unbreakable thread of fate that ties the journey of these planets together. We cannot speak about one without speaking about the other.

Frankly, a discussion on aspects in and of themselves could fill an entire book—and indeed, there are quite a few popular ones on exactly that! For the purposes of this book, however, and for brevity's sake, we will only be covering the most important and common ones here.

THE CONJUNCTION ☌

A conjunction occurs when two or more planets, points, or asteroids in the chart are within a few degrees of each other, often in the same sign. The number of degrees between the two planets—referred to as the "orb" in astrology—that determines whether or not they are conjunct varies among astrologers. However, the generally accepted range is within five degrees of each other. Essentially, the two heavenly bodies are right on top of, or next to, each other in the chart. This close-knit relationship creates a dynamic of incredible harmony within the chart—and therefore within that person's nature and their life. The two (or three, or four, etc.) planets, points, or asteroids want the same thing. They express themselves in the same way, through the same lens, and their journeys are inextricably tied together.

THE OPPOSITION ☍

The opposition is exactly what it sounds like. It's where two (or more) planets, points, or asteroids in the chart are directly opposite each other, sitting 180 degrees apart, give or take a few degrees. In this aspect, the cosmic spheres are (usually) in opposite signs and therefore are embodying two sides of the same coin. The opposition is a particularly interesting dynamic within the chart, as it can be both confusing/tense and harmonious/balancing. The very nature of an opposition puts the respective placements in a counterpoint position. Again, their journeys are inextricably linked, but until this dualistic nature is mastered by the individual, it can very much feel like a push and pull. The opposition is said to possess the nature of Saturn, which can help to explain the hard work involved in mastering this aspect, as well as the maturity that comes from doing so.

The flip side of this is that oppositions can also bring clarity and understanding, especially when the person is experiencing this aspect via a transit.

THE SQUARE □

In my opinion, the square in the natal chart is easily the most difficult dynamic one can have. A square aspect occurs between signs and planets that are 90 degrees apart, give or take a few degrees. Like the conjunction and the opposition, squares usually happen between signs of the same modality: cardinal, fixed, or mutable. The difference here is that there is a fundamental lack of harmony between the signs involved in a square. Just about the only thing they have in common is that they are the same modality and therefore possess the quintessential qualities of their respective category: Cardinal signs are leaders, fixed signs are tenacious, and mutable signs are adaptable. However, the similarities pretty much end there. The signs wrapped up in a square approach life in grossly different ways. This, too, creates a push-pull dynamic within a person.

The tension of a square can be incredibly dynamic and often leads us toward the most growth and evolution as we struggle to balance out these seemingly incompatible parts of ourselves and our lives. We have to work to make it work. Squares are said to possess the nature of Mars, which helps to describe the tension and conflict we often feel with these dynamics.

THE TRINE △

Trines usually occur in signs that share the same element: between water signs, earth signs, air signs, and fire signs, respectively. A trine aspect occurs between signs and planets that are 120 degrees apart, give or take a few degrees. A trine is a supportive aspect, taking on the nature of Jupiter, and is an expansive, easy connection. Just like with all other aspects, a trine between planets ties the journeys of those planets together, though it may not feel as strong as the other aspects we've already covered.

The exception to this, in my opinion, is when someone has a grand trine. This dynamic occurs when a person has a planet in all three signs of an element—Leo, Sagittarius, and Aries, for example—and those planets are in very close degrees, making aspects to each other. A grand trine is a powerful activation to have in a chart and places a special emphasis on the characteristics of the element the grand trine is made up of. Trines possess the nature of Jupiter, which speaks to the expansive, supportive, easy nature of this aspect.

THE SEXTILE ✳

The final aspect we'll cover here is the sextile, which occurs between signs and planets that are 60 degrees apart, give or take a few degrees. This aspect is said to possess the nature of Venus, again bringing a certain support and ease. Sextiles usually occur between supportive elements: fire and air or water and earth. There are lots of similarities between these two sets of signs, thus they come through to offer their subtle gifts to each other. The journeys of the two planets or points in the sextile are connected, as always, though less so than with the other aspects covered here.

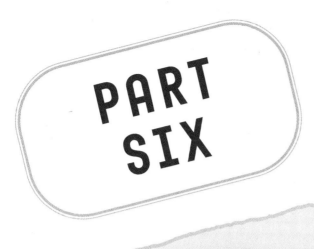

PART SIX

HOUSES

The twelve houses are the final key to understanding your sexual birth chart. The houses are a component that tends to be confusing for most people and is therefore usually the last frontier of exploration and understanding. That's okay—they can be a lot.

17
THE HOUSES

I would like to emphasize that all twelve houses in the chart matter. A common misconception that people have is that if a house doesn't contain any planets and is therefore "empty," it doesn't matter. While this assumption is understandable, it's simply not true. Rather, there is less of an emphasis on the themes of that house in your personal journey, but those themes are still there. For example, say you have an empty fourth house. This is the house of family, ancestors, roots, where you live, etc. Regardless of your personal circumstances with your family, we all have one! In fact, we would not exist without a family. You see what I mean?

Beyond this, it's important to understand that the birth chart is a mirror. The houses all exist in pairs and in relationship to each other. Thus, as you will soon see, I have chosen to write about them in terms of their respective pairings. I encourage you to familiarize yourself with all twelve houses to truly have a holistic understanding of yourself.

THE FIRST AND SEVENTH HOUSES

The axis of the first and seventh houses in the birth chart is the relationship axis. It's where we look at the self versus others and seek to achieve balance and harmony between the two.

The first house plays a very important role in the birth chart, whether looking at it through the lens of sextrology or just astrology in general. The cusp of the first house is known as the Ascendant and/or rising sign and is determined by the sign whose constellation was rising on the eastern horizon at the time you were born. This is why knowing your exact birth time is so important! It is *the* determining factor of the Ascendant, which then determines the entire layout of your chart. Without the correct time, everything gets screwed up really fast.

The first house has everything to do with our identity. It is the way we show up in the world. It is our beliefs and the face we readily wear and put forward and has a lot to do with the way we look. In short, the first house in the chart is the only house that's just you. Everything else is everything (and everyone) else, but the first house is solely you. Some people believe that the Ascendant is where the soul enters the body.

Everything that lies within the first house is up front for people to see. We readily embody the nature of any planet or asteroid in this house, and their energies have a great influence on who we are and how we present ourselves or identify. The closer a planet is to the actual degree of the Ascendant, the stronger the influence of that planet. For example, someone with Mars in the first house can be much more fiery and openly sexual than someone with their Mars hidden in the fourth. Planets in the first house can also influence the way we look. Someone with their Moon in the first house may have a round face, for example, or softer features, as opposed to Mars here, which may lend itself to sharper features. There are innumerable combinations and examples, and getting to know the ins and outs of your first house can help to weave together all the nuances of who you are.

The seventh house is the literal and figurative opposite of us: It is the house of others. The cusp of the seventh house is known as the Descendant. This house grapples with things like marriage, committed partnerships, and all our close, one-on-one intimate relationships, such as close friendships.

Generally speaking, the seventh house describes the characteristics we are attracted to where long-term relationships are concerned. Because of this, it's very common to end up with someone who has strong placements in the sign of your Descendant, though it isn't a guarantee. The sign on your seventh house can also describe the quality or nature of your serious relationships.

As an example, say you have Virgo on the cusp of your seventh house. This points to the desire to have a partner who is grounded, reliable, and very likely detail-oriented and who always has a plan of some sort. This is someone who is going to be oriented toward acts of service and embodies tangible acts of love that come from a place of wanting to help you. They may not be very touchy-feely and may even lean toward criticism, but their unwavering ability to show up and help you to ground yourself and your ideas feels like exactly what you need, as a Pisces rising, as you may feel like you struggle to find clarity, get organized, and nail things down. In that sense, as our Descendant is always in the opposite sign of our Ascendant, this is one way we can understand the age-old saying that opposites attract.

Any planets in your seventh house have an influence on the nature of your close relationships, too.

THE SECOND AND EIGHTH HOUSES

The second and eighth houses in the chart represent the axis of values and resources. It's also where we look at more surface-level relationships (such as acquaintances) versus the deep, intimate relationships in our lives.

In the natal chart, the second house represents our values. It's where we look at our own resources, which is to say our own money, assets, and the possessions or other things we have at our disposal, as well as our relationship to said resources. We seek material stability here, specifically the stability we are able to provide for ourselves. There is a journey around trusting our ability to take care of ourselves or to handle whatever may come our way in life thanks to our inherent resourcefulness.

We solidify the work we've done around our identity in the first house and therefore grapple with self-esteem in the second house. Especially through the lens of sextrology, this is the house of values. What do we value? Who do we value? And what value do we place on ourselves?

Because the second house is so focused on the material, it's also where we see our surface-level connections. Acquaintances fall in this house, as well as any relationships we have that are casual or don't go beyond the niceties.

The eighth house is the house of secrets, death, and sex, making it the most obvious place to look to when it comes to sextrology. This is a house of great depth, where we seek to constantly peel back the layers on someone, and ourselves, in order to foster both a physically intimate and an emotionally intimate connection that surpasses normal, everyday connections. This house is where we seek to have extraordinary experiences that surpass everyday, "normal" ones. It's here in the eighth house that we relentlessly excavate the superfluous in order to get to the heart of the matter and the person.

Similar to the journey of Pluto—and of Scorpio placements in general—the journey of the eighth house is cyclical. We come back to the things contained in our eighth house time and again, constantly going through the process of death, rebirth, and transformation. Even if this house is "empty," meaning there aren't any planets there, we still have a sign on the cusp of this house, and there's something about whatever that sign points to that we come back to over and over.

Say, for example, Taurus is on the cusp of your eighth house. First of all, you might be a person who is quite slow to embrace change in general, as Taurus is the sign that downright resists it. But where sex and intimacy are concerned, Taurus is incredibly sensual, perhaps even gluttonous, where matters of the flesh are concerned, preferring to take things slow and relish every sensation that is activated with skin on skin.

THE THIRD AND NINTH HOUSES

Moving on to the third and ninth houses, we look at the axis of communication and the big picture versus the finer details in life. Through the lens of sextrology, the ninth house is our overall beliefs or philosophy about love versus the way we execute that philosophy through all the minutiae in our interactions with others in the third house.

In the chart, the third house is often referred to as the house of the student. This makes sense when we consider the themes of this house, which include learning on a traditional level (such as reading) and communication. However, this house is also about short-term travel, our local environments, siblings, and, as mentioned above, the small picture/details.

As far as sextrology is concerned, the third house is truly the way we choose to share what we think and feel about love, romance, sex, and relationships as a whole. This house adds a layer of nuance to our Mercury placements in a way, especially if the two are in different signs. For example, someone with their Mercury in Sagittarius may want to spend time talking about their beliefs and exploring some of the headier questions when it comes to relationships. If they have Capricorn on the cusp of their third house, it will add a layer of groundedness and practical application to their beliefs, whereas if Pisces is on their third house cusp, their beliefs may be swept up in fantasy or idealism in some way. Exploring the connection between our Mercury placement and our third house can help us to really understand the way our mind works and how we express ourselves.

The ninth house, on the other hand, is known as the house of the teacher. It's here that we see things such as higher education, philosophy and ethics, the law, spirituality, religion, and dogma, as well as learning through experience. It's also where we see the big picture of our lives, as well as the topic of astrology!

Through the lens of sextrology, the ninth house is where we'll see someone's personal philosophy when it comes to sex. Because ethics is one of the themes of the ninth house, that gets tied in with our personal beliefs around love, romance, and sex as well. In short, this house points to what we believe in, in the grand scheme of things, when it comes to sexuality. These are things that we may believe to be objectively true, that transcend the boundaries of individuals, cultures, and societies and apply to humanity as a whole. As with every house, the sign on the cusp of the ninth house will largely influence our philosophy here, as will any of the points and planets that may reside here. For example, someone with their Sun in the ninth house may have a lot of their sexual identity rooted in what they believe is good and right and true, whereas someone with an empty ninth house may not identify with it so much, or perhaps they don't spend *so* much time and energy thinking about the larger questions when it comes to sex and ethics. I think it's important to spend some time exploring the nature of the ninth house and getting in touch with your own beliefs.

THE FOURTH AND TENTH HOUSES

In the fourth and tenth houses, we confront the axis of our most private self versus our most public self. These are the lowest and highest points in the chart, respectively, and make up the other set of "angles," just as the first and seventh houses make up the former set. I think it's important to consider these houses in sextrology, as they can greatly highlight the way other people perceive us in general and the way we feel inside, which can diverge quite a bit.

The fourth house is one of the most private places in the birth chart. The cusp of the fourth house is known as the *Imum Coeli*, or IC, and is the lowest point in the chart. The fourth house points to our families, foundations, ancestors, and roots. Similar to the second house, the fourth can also point to the actual space we live in: our house, apartment, condo, whatever. It is also our most private self, the person we are when nobody else is around.

There is a great deal that can be gleaned about a person by exploring the fourth house. The sign on the cusp of this house informs much about who we are when we're alone. In many ways, this may be the truest version of ourselves. It's the energy we embody when all our masks have been put down and we don't feel the need to perform or show up in any kind of way. Considering that the fourth is also the house of family, ideally those are the people we are our most natural self with, too (though I know that is far from the truth for plenty of people).

Regardless, our family and everything that entails has a huge influence on who we are. And if we end up in any kind of serious, long-term relationships, at some point we're probably going to introduce our partner to our family and vice versa. Understanding the dynamics, values, experiences, influences, and possible baggage that stem from the family of origin is important when it comes to both ourselves and our partners. The sign of the IC can reveal much about these themes.

Now, someone with a lot of planets in their fourth house can be both a very private, homebody type and a person who is greatly influenced by their family and perhaps quite family-oriented. An individual with their Sun here, for example, may like being at home. They may also want to be a parent themselves and build a family of their own someday. Perhaps they're very close with their family or their family's opinions hold a lot of weight with them. There are many possibilities.

As far as sex is concerned, someone with a lot of planets in the fourth house may be quite private or shy when it comes to sexual attention. They may not enjoy overt sexual attention from others, or perhaps they're just more reserved in this area, needing a solid foundation of safety and intimacy before being able to open up in that way.

The tenth house, unsurprisingly, is the exact opposite of the fourth. The cusp of the tenth house is known as the Midheaven, or MC, and is the highest point in the chart. The tenth house is our most public self and ultimately points to our calling in life. It's the work we are meant to do, the thing that fulfills us on a soul level. The meaning of the tenth house frequently gets reduced to the career, and while in an ideal world we would get paid to do the thing we love, I find that meaning to be highly reductive. Sometimes the purpose we're here to fulfill has nothing to do with work. And in our highly capitalistic society, that description so often reduces us to how productive we are. I think it's of the utmost importance to remember that.

That said, our tenth house is the face the public or community at large sees. In that sense I think there's a similarity between the tenth and the first houses. Both have a lot to do with the way we present ourselves, and anything contained in these houses is up front for people to see. The difference is that whereas the first house is personal, the tenth house happens on a much higher and broader scale. We are highly visible in the tenth house—it's truly how we are perceived by the general public.

When thinking about this dynamic through the lens of sextrology, its meaning maybe doesn't feel so obvious. I think a great example of this would be someone who has their Venus or Mars in the tenth but their Moon in the fourth. Generally speaking, this would be someone others see as beautiful and sensual and possibly find quite sexually attractive, but with their Moon in the fourth, the person may actually not feel safe being perceived that way.

THE FIFTH AND ELEVENTH HOUSES

In the fifth and eleventh houses, we look at the axis of the individual versus the group. The fifth house is all about us as individuals: how we express ourselves, find joy, and live in the moment. The eleventh house, on the other hand, asks us about the community we belong to. Through the lens of sextrology, this could be things like a kink community, for example.

The fifth is the house of pleasure. Its main themes are fun, joy, play, romance, children, and the present moment. It's important to note that when we speak of romance in the fifth house, we are talking about casual relationships. This is the house of hookups, summer flings (or any fling for that matter), situationships, and one-night stands. Similar to the seventh house, the sign on the cusp of the fifth house can indicate the people we're attracted to, albeit casually—at least at first. This doesn't mean you are doomed to only have casual connections with those of whatever sign is on this house cusp, but there may be a disproportionate number when it comes to the sign you hook up with a lot. The sign on the cusp of the fifth house can also color your approach to romance in general.

Both casual relationships and children are associated with the fifth house, and personally I find the combination to be a strange one. Again we see an influence via the sign on this house cusp to speak to our views on children. Someone with Cancer on the cusp of their fifth house may be all about children, for example, whereas someone with an Aquarius fifth house may not be interested in them at all or may want to adopt instead of having their own. Now, I want to underline that we all have free will, and nothing in the chart dooms you to having kids or not. This is merely one factor to consider. Keep in mind, too, that we can see our own inner child here, as well as the things in our life that we wish to birth, nurture, or manifest.

The fifth house is also where we explore our relationship to pleasure and fun. Again, the sign on the cusp of the fifth house, as well as any planets that may be here, can inform us about the activities we find enjoyable. Having Uranus in the fifth, for example, can point to someone who is a bit of a daredevil or derives pleasure from unexpected avenues.

The eleventh house, on the other hand, is the house of community. It is where all our various social circles exist: friends, family, lovers, neighbors, coworkers. It's all the people we interact with on a regular basis, if not daily. It's also the house of the future, our hopes and dreams, social justice, and technology.

Now, when speaking about the eleventh house through the lens of sextrology, we are looking at potential communities we may be involved in or could benefit from joining. One example, of course, is the kink community. Kink shows up in too many ways to name here, but maybe you love shibari or BDSM or whatever. Having Saturn, the planet of bondage, in the eleventh is a great example. Sometimes astrology can be quite literal.

Another example of community could be the queer community, or the sexual health community, or a poly group. Again, the sign on the cusp of eleventh house can shed light on the possibilities. Any planets contained herein can also reveal a great deal about a person's relationship to community and the group in general. For example, someone with their Venus in the eleventh house may often meet lovers through friends or other people they know. People with their South Node in the eleventh may struggle greatly with community and are actually being asked to focus more on themselves in this lifetime. Someone with their Pluto in the eleventh will have a lot of karma to work out where the group is concerned, and so on.

Outside of this, we also look at our hopes, dreams, and vision for the future in the eleventh house. This house paves the way for the future and asks us about our wishes: What do we want for ourselves? Who do we want to be there? And so on.

THE SIXTH AND TWELFTH HOUSES

The the sixth and twelfth are the final pair of houses in the chart. These houses grapple with health, both mental and physical, as well as the spiritual and the mundane. Through the sexual lens we can see how we're taking care of ourselves and how we're showing up in real time in our day-to-day lives versus the escapism and fantasy we may tend to live in.

As the sixth house represents our physical health, I find it to be extremely important. In our modern age of casual sex, taking our sexual health into account is more important—and possible—than ever before. In sextrology, it is in this house in particular that we can see a person's approach to and values surrounding health. The sixth house reveals a person's approach to health overall, as well as how they take care of themselves in the day-to-day. Understanding this house is crucial where sextrology is concerned. It is impossible, in my opinion, to overstate the importance of good sexual hygiene and overall wellness. The most fulfilling sex lives are built upon a foundation of good practices. Someone with a lot of planets—or truly any planets—in the sixth house is going to take their health, as well as their partners' health, quite seriously.

Outside of this, the sixth house points to our everyday, mundane lives. It's where we see our daily routines and rituals, our job, and our pets. The sign on the cusp of the sixth house describes the energy we bring to our daily lives and health matters. For example, someone with Aries on the cusp of their sixth house likely has a ton of energy to burn and would benefit greatly from having an exercise routine or playing sports. Keep in mind that no matter which sign is on your sixth house cusp, it's important for all of us to exercise and move the body somehow. The sign of this area of the chart can also point to the types of exercise a person enjoys. Someone with Aries on the cusp of their sixth house might enjoy something competitive or independently paced. Someone with Pisces on their sixth house cusp might enjoy swimming or dancing, and so on. Someone with a lot of planets in the sixth house will take their health and job quite seriously. They will likely be very busy people.

Conversely, the final house in the birth chart, the twelfth, is a very curious place indeed. As the only house in the chart that never sees the light of day from the Sun, it is completely shrouded in obscurity. Because of this, it is, in my opinion, the most misunderstood house of the bunch.

Ultimately, the twelfth house represents the subconscious mind. Everything contained herein is happening just under the surface of our conscious awareness, which helps to explain why this house is so confusing. We have to work extra hard to engage with everything happening here.

We all have parts of ourselves that we struggle to understand, and thus we may spend our entire lives engaging with these pieces of our lives time and again in order to flesh them out. In order to do that, we need solitude, peace, quiet, time, and space to engage with whatever this final house is asking of us. People who have placements in the twelfth house require a lot of alone time. However, even if you don't have any planets here, it's important to note that an "empty" twelfth house still has one of the signs on its cusp. None of us escape the journey of this final space.

The twelfth house asks us to look at our mental health as well as our tendency to escape reality. Just as physical health is important where sex is concerned, mental health is too.

The uniqueness of romance inevitably finds us having to deal with feelings we've never experienced before—good, bad, and ugly—and if you've been dating long enough, you will eventually experience heartbreak in some way, which in turn will affect your mental health. Having the right tools and coping mechanisms is of the utmost importance, and there's much that can be revealed to us about our needs and tendencies in this area by studying the twelfth house. I think it's also important to understand that we tend to repress and bury things in this house. A lot of us have locked our issues away at one point or another instead of dealing with them in a healthy way, and the place where we locked them away is in this final house. I strongly encourage all of you to understand the twelfth house as best you can. It will help you in more than just romance and sex.

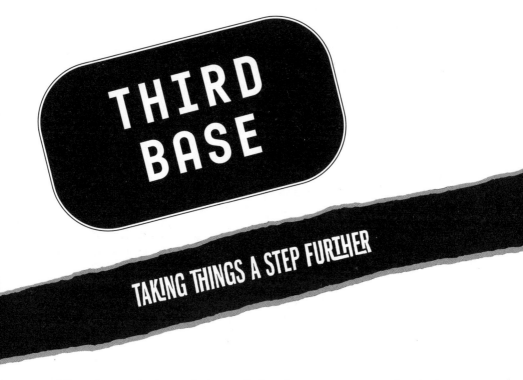

THIRD BASE

TAKING THINGS A STEP FURTHER

Now that you've learned about all the placements in your chart, what do you *do* with this information? Well, the first step is to put them all together.

Now that you've read through each section and have a better understanding of what each of your natal placements means and looks like, spend some time exploring how and where and when you experience them and embody them. Tangible examples of astrology are incredibly important, and being able to point to and name moments or feelings helps us get a better grasp of the role a placement plays in our lives. Being able to take the time to piece together how we feel we embody each planet, asteroid, or point can help us weave together a cohesive picture around the true nature of our erotic self and just what it is, exactly, that we're hunting for.

Keep in mind it's highly possible that some of your placements may seem to contradict or be at odds with each other. Having a Pisces Venus that desires deep emotional connections and is highly

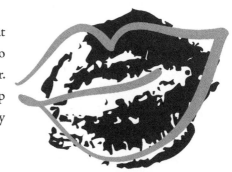

sensitive paired with a Gemini Mars that is fun and flirty and wants variety in sex and sexual partners is just one example. It is just as common as it is uncommon to experience things like this. The makeup of our charts is highly complex and nuanced, just like relationships, just like being a person. It's true that having these push-pull dynamics within ourselves makes things feel complicated. We may end up feeling like we have to choose one or the other, or that we don't understand these parts of ourselves that seem to contradict each other. This is normal. However, that doesn't necessarily mean it's right.

On the contrary, this is an invitation for you to hold space for all the weird, wonderful, and diverse parts of yourself. You can wish to have both fun and deep connections. You can want variety and commitment, or a grounded yet casual partner. There are an impossible number of combinations and intersections that exist across humanity, and I promise that just as you are more than one thing, there are other people out there who are made up just as strangely and brilliantly as you are.

Which brings us to our next step: applying what you've learned in real relationships.

The very point of engaging with the exploration of the self, and gleaning whatever knowledge and wisdom we can, is to enable ourselves to take what we know and apply it to our real lives. Without the actual, tangible follow-through, it makes everything we've gained morph a moot point. It's okay if it feels awkward or scary or intimidating or exciting or whatever at first—that's normal. But without actual application and practice, we're not going to get what we want. As they say, nothing changes if nothing changes.

Maybe the easiest way to begin making the changes you desire is to explore this book with your partner(s) and learn about yourselves together. An inevitable part of this process involves communicating your wants, needs, and desires. At some point you're going to have to speak up for yourself, but maybe having a resource that explains it for you will be helpful at first. Plus, it can be a fun way to learn more about each other.

THE PROGRESSED SEXUAL CHART

We will end our journey with sextrology with a final note on seeing how our sexual expression transforms over time. Just as we grow, evolve, and change throughout life, our birth chart does too. We can track the changes in our chart—and therefore the various cycles in our lives and changes within ourselves—through a technique in astrology known as secondary progressions.

This is a timing technique that takes the varying transits of the planets in the first ninety days after we're born and applies one day to one year of life. So the first day is the first year of our lives, the second day is the second year, the thirtieth day is year thirty, and so on. Every time a planet changes signs and/or houses in our chart, it signals a change both within us and in the external circumstances of our lives. In my own practice, I've found it to be an insightful exercise to apply this same technique to the sexual birth chart.

CONCLUSION

The different experiences we have in our romantic and sexual encounters greatly inform what we know about our true needs and desires and cause those things to change across time. What we need in our thirties is different from what we need in our twenties, and what we need in our forties and fifties is even more different from what we need as teens and young adults. This same growth is reflected in our progressed charts as our natal placements shift over the course of our lives. While we are always, at our core, the person with the placements we were born with, the progressions of the planets add an extra layer of nuance and complexity. In many ways, our natal charts are simply the starting line. For example, say someone has their natal Venus in Sagittarius, but at some point in their thirties their Venus progresses into Capricorn. That person will still value their independence and want a partner who wants to go out and do things together—to experience all that life has to offer together—but now they feel more serious about committing to someone and finding a partner who shares the same values. They may start to feel more serious about settling down, as opposed to being more averse to such things, as Sagittarius can be prone to.

Now, how and when things progress from one chart to another depends entirely on your subjective placements. Just as the planets move at different speeds through the signs, progressions move at different speeds as well. Because of this, we mostly look to the progressed personal planets—Sun, Moon, Mercury, Venus, and Mars, as well as the Ascendant—and not so much anything outside of that. Of course, there are rare exceptions where someone's Saturn or Pluto or lunar nodes can change signs, but they are few and far between. However, should your Venus or Mars change signs, for example, you can expect that the way you show up in your relationships, as well as the way you express yourself sexually and romantically, will change too.

Just like aspects in the chart, progressions alone could easily fill an entire book. However, finding out where your current progressions are is just as easy as pulling up your birth chart. The internet is a beautiful thing. A simple search will bring up plenty of free databases where you can access your progressed charts. Once you have that information available, I recommend going back through the book and reading for your progressed placements as well. They may ring truer than you expect.

ACKNOWLEDGMENTS

I would first like to express my gratitude to Amy Glaser and the entire team at Llewellyn, as well as Adriana Stimola, for immediately seeing and understanding the vision of this book and enthusiastically embracing it. It is because of them that this book was able to come into existence.

Second, I would like to acknowledge my dear friend Anthony Perrotta for his tireless consultation and patience with helping me flesh out all my ideas. You are an invaluable well of knowledge, love, and friendship. This book would not be what it is without your help.

And finally, to everyone who chooses to pick up a copy of this book, from the bottom of my heart, thank you.

TO WRITE TO THE AUTHOR

If you wish to contact the author or would like more information about this book, please write to the author in care of Llewellyn Worldwide Ltd. and we will forward your request. Both the author and the publisher appreciate hearing from you and learning of your enjoyment of this book and how it has helped you. Llewellyn Worldwide Ltd. cannot guarantee that every letter written to the author can be answered, but all will be forwarded. Please write to:

Aubrey Houdeshell
⁒ Llewellyn Worldwide
2143 Wooddale Drive
Woodbury, MN 55125-2989

Please enclose a self-addressed stamped envelope for reply,
or $1.00 to cover costs. If outside the U.S.A., enclose
an international postal reply coupon.

Many of Llewellyn's authors have websites with additional information and resources. For more information, please visit our website at http://www.llewellyn.com.